Neurovirology

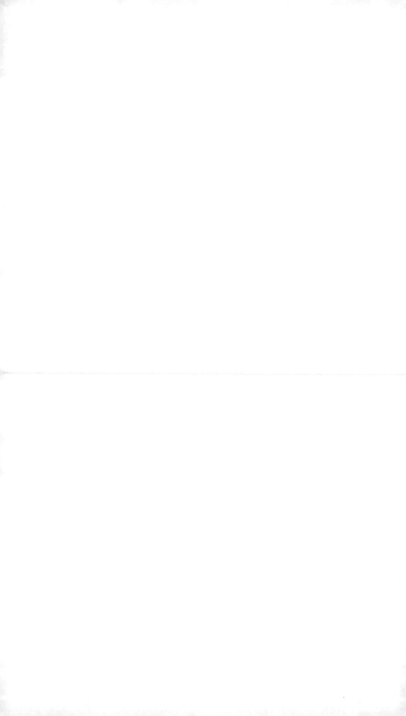

Neurovirology

Measuring, Interpreting, and Understanding Viruses

Richard B. Tenser, MD, MS
Deposit, New York, USA
Professor Emeritus, Penn State University, State College, Pennsylvania, USA
Former Professor of Neurology, Penn State University College of Medicine,
Hershey, Pennsylvania, USA
Former Professor of Microbiology and Immunology, Penn State University
College of Medicine, Hershey, Pennsylvania, USA

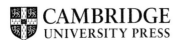
CAMBRIDGE
UNIVERSITY PRESS

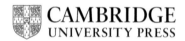

University Printing House, Cambridge CB2 8BS, United Kingdom

One Liberty Plaza, 20th Floor, New York, NY 10006, USA

477 Williamstown Road, Port Melbourne, VIC 3207, Australia

314–321, 3rd Floor, Plot 3, Splendor Forum, Jasola District Centre,
New Delhi – 110025, India

103 Penang Road, #05–06/07, Visioncrest Commercial, Singapore 238467

Cambridge University Press is part of the University of Cambridge.

It furthers the University's mission by disseminating knowledge in the pursuit of
education, learning, and research at the highest international levels of excellence.

www.cambridge.org
Information on this title: www.cambridge.org/9781009235556
DOI: 10.1017/9781009235563

First published 2023

Printed in the United Kingdom by CPI Group Ltd, Croydon CR0 4YY

A catalogue record for this publication is available from the British Library.

ISBN 978-1-009-23555-6 Paperback

For Janet

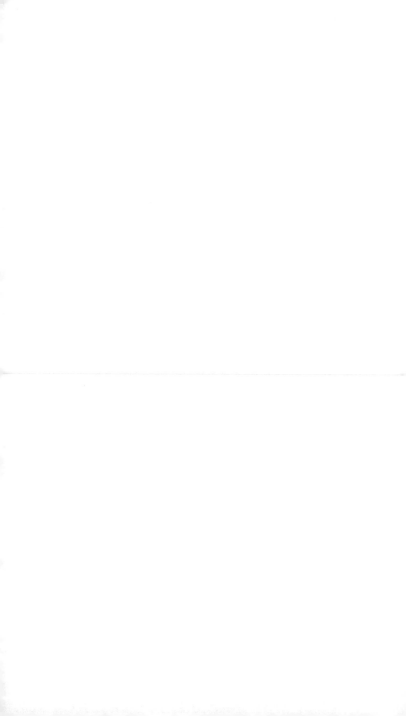

Contents

Preface   *page* ix

1 Introduction to Virology   1

2 Measurement of Infectious Virus   34

3 Molecular Biology: The Synthesis of DNA,
   RNA, Protein   45

4 The Immune System: Innate and Adaptive   68

5 Viral Pathogenesis   94

6 Viral Infections of the Nervous System   122

7 Neurovirology and Immunology   142

8 Experimental Neurovirology   180

9 The Future   194

References   206
Index   213

Preface

Interest in virology has increased greatly due to the recent COVID-19 pandemic, caused by the coronavirus given the name SARS-CoV-2. An initial impetus to write this book was related to reports that the COVID-19 virus could "live" for days on hard surfaces. The nucleic acid of SARS-CoV-2, its RNA, might be detected on a park bench, but did that mean that living virus was present? Even if viruses could live on surfaces (are viruses living things?), the important issue is whether they are infectious.

In addition, there continues to be much interest in viral and inflammatory illnesses of the nervous system. This includes viral infections of the nervous system, and also inflammatory illnesses of the nervous system that might be triggered by viral infections, including multiple sclerosis and Guillain–Barré syndrome. Related to these illnesses is the concept of latent virus infections and how these differ from acute and persistent viral infections.

A side point of emphasis in this book is on the interpretation of scientific and medical results. In brief, there is a difference between results (data) and the interpretation of that data. For example, does the polymerase chain reaction (PCR) detection of SARS-CoV-2 RNA on a surface (data) indicate the presence of "living" virus (interpretation of data)?

Some of the many known viruses are human pathogens. On the other hand, some viruses (endogenous retroviruses) seem to be part of the human genome, that is part of our DNA. These and other replicating agents such as viroids and prions may need be considered more in terms of human biology than in terms of human infections. Prion diseases of the nervous system are striking in that these illnesses can be genetically transmitted but are also infectious. But prions are proteins and contain no RNA or DNA.

After initial discussions of virology, including methods to measure and count infectious virus particles (Chapters 1, 2), an introduction to aspects molecular biology follows (Chapter 3). This introduces discussion of how viruses replicate, and also methods of nucleic acid detection such as PCR methodology. Discussion includes the conversion of nucleosides into nucleotides, important in considering nucleoside analogues as antivirals.

Discussions of immunology follow (Chapter 4). Included are discussions of the roles of the innate immune system (for example, cytokines) and the acquired immune system (lymphocytes and antibody). Considerations of the clinical use of antibody, including monoclonal antibody (passive immunization), lead to discussions of the use of vaccines (active immunization).

Chapters that emphasize basic science virology are followed by Chapter 5 on viral pathogenesis, important in understanding how illnesses occur. The concepts of slow and latent virus infections are discussed, with particular emphasis on infections of the nervous system. It is noted that latent virus infections are present in most humans. Viral illnesses of humans are presented, with emphasis on infections of the nervous system (Chapter 6).

Chapter 7 on neurovirology follows. Discussion emphasizes illnesses caused by viruses and atypical agents, and also inflammatory-demyelinating illnesses of the nervous system, including Guillain-Barré syndrome and multiple sclerosis. Guillain-Barré syndrome is an illness of the peripheral nervous system (PNS) and multiple sclerosis (MS) an illness of the central nervous system (CNS). Differences between the PNS and the CNS are discussed.

Following the more clinical discussions in Chapters 6 and 7 is discussion of experimental neurovirology (Chapter 8), particularly latent herpes simplex virus (HSV) infection of the nervous system. This expands on the pathogenesis discussions of Chapter 5. Emphasis includes the role of the nucleoside thymidine and how it may be of importance in latent HSV infection of neurons.

Chapter 9 is devoted to the discussion of possible future developments in virology and neurovirology.

As a Neurologist and Virologist, the author thought he could provide a somewhat unique perspective to some illnesses caused by viruses, including human latent virus infections.

Introduction to Virology

The COVID-19 pandemic caused by the virus SARS-CoV-2 has greatly increased interest in virology. The following chapters build on that interest.

Chapter 1 provides an overview of virology, including discussions of the detection of viruses. Chapter 2 focuses further on those discussions, and assays to specifically measure infectious virus particles are presented. Chapter 3 includes discussions of some aspects of molecular biology, important in considering the replication of viruses and the mechanisms of antiviral medications. Discussion of immunology, important in considering host mechanisms to control virus infections, follows in Chapter 4. Chapter 5 discusses viral pathogenesis, particularly infection of the nervous system. Chapters 6 and 7 discuss viral and immune-mediated illnesses of the nervous system. Chapter 8 discusses experimental neurovirology, and Chapter 9 looks at possible future aspects of virology and neurovirology.

What Are Viruses?

Viruses are very simple organisms that may infect people, animals, plants, and even bacteria. Specific viruses infect only specific types of animals, plants, and bacteria. Most of the known viruses do not infect humans. Recent epidemics and pandemics due to viruses such as human immunodeficiency disease virus (HIV), influenza virus, Ebola virus, Zika virus, West Nile virus, recently SARS-CoV-2, and most recently mpox virus (formerly monkeypox) have emphasized human viral infections. Many people are concerned about the development of new viruses that might infect humans. Viruses are not inhibited by antibiotics, which inhibit bacteria, but they may be inhibited by antiviral medications. Recent antiviral medication development has emphasized treatment of HIV infections, the cause of acquired immunodeficiency disease syndrome (AIDS).

Viral infections may be asymptomatic. That is, testing the blood serum of some people shows the presence of antibody to a virus, indicating prior infection, although those people do not have a clear history of clinically apparent infection by the virus.

Are Viruses Alive?

Are viruses living organisms? This will depend in large part on how one defines living organisms. Discussion of this point starts here with viruses and later moves to discussion of even simpler atypical agents.

Some may consider viruses as living organisms, although many would not. An initial conclusion is that infections may be caused not only by bacteria and fungi, which are living organisms, but also by viruses and atypical agents, which are not living organisms.

Viruses consist of a nucleic acid (RNA or DNA) core and viral proteins, and some (including SARS-CoV-2) have a lipid envelope containing additional viral proteins, such as the "spike" proteins of SARS-CoV-2. Viruses are classified as being either RNA viruses (SARS-CoV-2, polio, mumps, measles, influenza, HIV) or DNA viruses (herpes simplex, chickenpox, smallpox, papilloma). Some DNA viruses contain a single strand of DNA (these viruses are uncommon) or they contain double-stranded DNA (more common). RNA viruses contain double-stranded RNA (these viruses are uncommon) or they contain a single strand of RNA (more common). The viral RNA or DNA nucleic acid (the viral genome) is the substrate for viral reproduction and the synthesis of new viral RNA or DNA. The viral genome is also the blueprint for the synthesis of viral proteins.[1]

Viruses can readily reproduce. If one starts with 100 infectious virus particles and places them on living cells that are susceptible to them and keeps them at body temperature, in a few days there will be many more virus particles. Important words in this sentence include "infectious" (not all virus particles are infectious); "living cells" (viruses can only reproduce in living cells); "that are susceptible to them" (specific viruses only infect certain cell types, for example, skin cells but not blood cells, and cells from some animals, for example, mice or humans, but not others). Viruses are obligate intracellular organisms and only grow (replicate) inside of cells.

Bacteria such as rickettsia are also obligate intracellular organisms. However, unlike viruses they may be considered as living organisms, in large part because they replicate by fission. Viruses may be thought of as reproducing but not living organisms. The concept of agents that reproduce but are not living organisms is discussed further in considering atypical agents such as prions.

Infection of specific cell type(s) by a virus is sometimes termed the tropism of that virus. This is somewhat implied for SARS-CoV-2 when discussing it as causing respiratory infections. Later discussion includes poliomyelitis virus, which causes clinical polio by infecting specific cell types in the spinal cord. Some viruses have narrow tropisms, and some infect many cell types.

Many virus particles are not infectious. In Chapter 2 (viral plaque assay), discussion of how infectious virus particles may be measured (counted) is presented. Infectious and noninfectious virus particles may appear similar when examined by electron microscopy (discussed below). Polymerase chain reaction (PCR) technology, which is commonly used to detect viral nucleic acid, does not differentiate between infectious and noninfectious virus.

Reports in the news stating that SARS-CoV-2 can "live" for several days on hard surfaces (for example, a bench) are probably not accurate, in that the investigators did not determine the presence of infectious virus. It is assumed that when people discuss "live" virus, they mean infectious virus. However, the reports that live virus was detected usually relied on PCR methods that detected part of the virus (some of its RNA) but not the entire viral RNA genome. The entire viral genome is necessary for virus replication. As noted above, the genome of an organism is all of the nucleic acid, DNA or RNA, by which a virus reproduces copies of itself.

PCR technology is introduced below and discussed in detail in Chapter 3.

Virus Infection and Replication

Viruses can only reproduce in living cells, and they use the cellular biochemistry to reproduce. In describing clinical or experimental situations wherein virus numbers are increased, the terms "reproduce," "grow," "replicate" will be used interchangeably. The fact that viruses only grow in living cells is one reason it has been difficult to develop antiviral medications: inhibition of viral growth may also inhibit the functions of the cells in which they are growing.

Most investigations of virus infections of cells have been performed in cell culture, in living cells cultivated in the laboratory, that is, in vitro. Cell culture is discussed further in Chapter 2. In vivo studies refer to those in intact living individuals (animals or people).

Viruses get into cells (necessary if the virus is to reproduce) by an active process. Viruses do not simply infect all cells that they contact. Typically, part(s) of the virus (for example, a specific protein on its surface) binds to a specific cell protein on the cell surface. If cells do not have the specific protein "recognized" by the virus protein, the virus will not bind to the cell, will not enter the cell, and will not infect the cell. Some cells of the human upper respiratory tract have the cell surface protein to which, for example, SARS-CoV-2 spikes bind. These viral spikes can be visualized (by electron microscopy) on the surface of SARS-CoV-2 particles. The receptor on human cells to which SARS-CoV-2 spikes bind is the human cell surface angiotensin-converting enzyme (ACE) protein.

To date, there has not been evidence of an effect of ACE inhibitors or ACE receptor blockers, commonly used to treat hypertension, on COVID-19, caused by SARS-CoV-2.

Transfection

Although the matching of a viral protein and a cell receptor protein noted above are the usual means by which viruses bind to cells, following which viral nucleic acid is introduced into the cells, mention should be made of a process by which viral nucleic acid is directly entered into cells. Termed "transfection," this is an experimental process by which viral nucleic acid is directly introduced into cells.[2] By this process, it is possible to have viral nucleic acid enter cells without the more typical infection sequence of events. Viral transfection procedures have been used in investigations of viral transformation of cells to investigate possible viral causes of cancer.

Viruses are thought to cause cancer by having their nucleic acid inserted into the DNA of the host cells. Viruses that may cause cancer in humans include Epstein-Barr virus, hepatitis B virus, hepatitis C virus, human herpesvirus type 8, human papillomavirus, and human T-lymphotropic virus type 1. In addition, HIV, an RNA virus, may cause AIDS, and people with this illness are at increased risk for several types of cancer, related to their immunosuppression.

Infection

Returning to consideration of the process of viral infection of cells, investigations have focused on cell surface proteins. Cell surface proteins to which viruses bind vary very much among cell types (muscle cells, skin cells, and blood cells) of an individual and among cells of different animals. Similarly, the proteins on the surface of viruses vary greatly. When there is a match, that is, when the virus protein (for example, the spikes on SARS-CoV-2) are able to bind to protein on the cell surface (for example, ACE), the virus enters and infects the cell.

Once inside the cell, there must also be a match whereby the viral nucleic acid (RNA in the case of SARS-CoV-2) can interact with and use the cellular biochemistry to reproduce itself. Virus-infected cells are usually destroyed during this process. However, some viruses establish latent infections, whereby destructive viral effects may be slight. These cells appear to continue their usual functions, and the virus is maintained in the cell. However, in most instances, virus-infected cells are destroyed.

Infections in which the infected host cells are destroyed are termed "lytic infections" (the infected cells are lysed) to differentiate them from latent infections in which the infected cells appear not to be damaged. Some viruses, for example, HIV and herpes simplex virus (HSV), cause both lytic and latent infections (Chapter 5).

Some viruses infect bacteria, and the occurrence of such viral infections has led to considerations of viruses as therapeutic agents. For example, bacteriophages, viruses that specifically infect bacteria, have been considered as therapeutic agents, using viruses to destroy bacteria.

In further consideration of "therapeutic" viruses, oncolytic viruses, viruses that infect and kill cancer cells, have been considered. And viruses have been used to transport DNA genes into individuals with genetic illnesses. These "therapeutic" viral options are discussed later in this chapter and in Chapter 9.

Infectious Virus vs Living Virus

Viruses are not alive, and it is probably not an important discussion point; rather, whether a virus is infectious or not is the important point. It is stretch to conclude that viruses are ever "alive," and most investigators would probably conclude they are not.

The important question is whether a virus is infectious. The reports that SARS-CoV-2 can "live" on surfaces for days, that is, viral RNA was detected by PCR (polymerase chain reaction) methodology, do not enhance understanding of whether it is infectious. However, they may be important in considering SARS-CoV-2 epidemiology, and the spread of the virus (Epidemiology is discussed below).

Detection of Virus by PCR

It is possible to use PCR technology to detect the DNA of DNA viruses, and, with slightly increased complexity, the RNA of RNA viruses. PCR techniques greatly increase the amount of target nucleic acid, for example, SARS-CoV-2 RNA, facilitating its detection. PCR methodology is more thoroughly discussed in Chapter 3.

PCR studies of SARS-CoV-2 virus RNA almost always investigate the presence of only part of the viral RNA genome. And even if the entire viral RNA were present (the entire genome), it would not necessarily mean that infectious virus was present – for infectious virus to be present, the protein spikes in the viral envelope and other viral factors would also need to be present. These are not detected by PCR methodology.

By analogy, the presence at a site of all of the DNA of a human cell (the entire human genome) would not necessarily indicate that a living cell is present.

PCR Data and Its Interpretation

Polymerase chain reaction technology has been the most widely used technology in reports of SARS-CoV-2, noting the presence of viral RNA. Many sites have been sampled, including throat swabs (nasopharyngeal swabs) and park benches. The possible presence of all of the viral nucleic acid could be investigated by PCR methodology, but most PCR studies only determine the presence of a small amount of viral nucleic acid to conclude that the virus is present. In the case of SARS-CoV-2, PCR has usually been performed to detect 2 or 3 of the probably 29 RNA genes of the virus.

The presence of SARS-CoV-2 RNA by PCR in a swab – from a nasopharyngeal or from a park bench swab – is the data (the result of a test) that indicates that the viral genome was present (at least part of the viral genome was present). The interpretation of that data, whether it indicates the presence of infectious virus, would remain to be determined.

After a digression to discuss the interpretation of data, for example, PCR data, methods other than PCR to detect viruses is then presented.

Data vs the Interpretation of Data: Results vs the Interpretation of Results

Relative to the detection of SARS-CoV-2 RNA and whether that suggests infectious virus is present, a brief discussion is presented to consider data versus the interpretation of data. For example, if viral RNA is present (data), is infectious virus present (interpretation of the data)? One could directly determine the presence of infectious virus (data), as in Chapter 2, but when PCR methods are used to detect virus, positive results (data) require an additional step to consider whether infectious virus is present.

The detection of SARS-CoV-2 RNA by PCR technology in a throat or nasopharyngeal swab of an individual very likely does indicate the presence of infectious virus. The PCR detection of the viral RNA in such swabs (data) does not prove the presence of infectious virus, but it can very reasonably be concluded that it indicates the presence of infectious virus (the interpretation of the data). Since the throat or nasopharyngeal swab was from a living individual and includes human throat or nasal epithelial cells where the virus likely grew, it is very reasonable to conclude that infectious virus is present.

However, it is not likely that the same detection of SARS-CoV-2 RNA from a park bench using PCR technology could be similarly interpreted. It is very unlikely that intact living throat or other human cells are present in the bench-positive swab. Even if the whole viral RNA genome were detected (not usually determined in most PCR studies), it could not be concluded that infectious virus is present. To be infectious, SARS-CoV-2 particles would need viral proteins and lipid, in addition to RNA.

Second, some PCR-testing results raise another interesting issue of data interpretation – whether all SARS-CoV-2–positive PCR nasopharyngeal swab results, which do suggest the presence of infectious virus (data), should be interpreted as indicating that the clinical illness COVID-19 is present (interpretation of data). Some people with SARS-CoV-2–positive swabs do not have clinical evidence of any illness, and illness is usually considered to exist in individuals with symptoms. Despite not having symptoms, these PCR-positive individuals (data) are usually counted as cases of COVID-19 (interpretation of data). The issue of SARS-CoV-2–positive throat swabs in asymptomatic individuals and whether this should be interpreted as indicating the presence of illness (COVID-19) is further considered below in discussions of epidemiology.

Data and the Interpretation of Data

In science and medicine there is data (results) and the interpretation of the data. PCR results indicating the presence of SARS-CoV-2 RNA in a nasopharyngeal swab from an individual are reasonably interpreted as indicating the presence of infectious virus. The detection of that the same piece of viral RNA on a park bench should likely not be similarly interpreted.

Methods to Detect Viruses

To return to methods to detect viruses, in addition to PCR, multiple other methods exist for the detection of viruses.

THE DETECTION OF VIRAL DNA OR RNA

Multiple molecular methods have been used to detect viral DNA or RNA as means to identify the specific causes of viral infections. Recently, PCR methods have been the most popular. Historically, PCR was preceded by Southern (DNA) and northern (RNA) methods – which were primarily used in research studies. Newer methods that might supplant PCR are being developed.

Most recent are metagenomic next-generation sequencing (mNGS) methods to determine the presence of the nucleic acids of viruses and other pathogens.

These molecular biology methods rely on the concepts of complementary DNA and RNA, and secondly on the hybridization of complementary DNA and RNA.

As discussed in Chapter 3, specific sequences of DNA will hybridize (bind to) other specific sequences of DNA to which they are complementary. They will also bind to complementary sequences of RNA. If a specific DNA sequence (the probe) is labeled, when it binds to (hybridizes with) a specific viral DNA or RNA (the target), the label will provide evidence for the presence of the specific target DNA or RNA virus.

Southern and Northern Blot Hybridization to Detect Viral DNA and RNA, Respectively

The first of the blot hybridization techniques to be developed was the use of a labeled DNA probe to detect target DNA, described by Edwin Southern. Therefore, the technique has often been described as a "Southern blot" study. When DNA probes were subsequently used to

Table 1.1 Blot hybridization

Target*	Southern blot DNA	Northern blot RNA
Procedure	Electrophoresis of the target in an agarose gel**	
Additional step	Denaturation of DNA***	None
Blot of gel after electrophoresis	DNA or RNA in the gel is transferred to a nylon membrane	
Probe	Single-stranded DNA complementary to the DNA or the RNA target, labeled with a radioactive or chemical tag****	
Detection of target	Sites of radioactive signal or of chemical color on the membrane where the probe which was complementary to the target and therefore hybridized to the target indicates the location of the target DNA or RNA*****	

*   Tissue containing the target DNA or RNA is homogenized and prepared.

**   DNA and RNA fragments move at different speeds in the gel, based on their sizes.

***   DNA is double stranded (the double-stranded helix), discussed in Chapter 3. For study, the DNA is denatured – the double strands are separated into two single strands. RNA is single stranded, and so this step is not needed.

**** A single-stranded fragment of DNA (probe) that is complementary to single-stranded DNA or RNA (target) will hybridize (bind to) the target.

***** Complementation and hybridization are discussed in Chapter 3.

detect RNA, the technique was termed a northern blot study (Table 1.1). In recent years, PCR methodology has replaced blot hybridization in many situations. The former is considerably less labor intensive than the latter.

In many ways, the concepts of Southern and northern blot hybridization are similar, whereby labeled DNA probes are used to bind to complementary target DNA (Southern) or RNA (northern).

DNA hybridization that detected human polyoma virus DNA in the brain of a patient with the illness progressive multifocal leukoencephalopathy (PML) is shown in Chapter 7.

THE DETECTION OF VIRAL PROTEINS (ANTIGENS)

As discussed in Chapter 4, antibodies bind to specific proteins (antigens). If such antibody is labeled, when it binds to a specific viral antigen, the label will provide evidence for the presence of the virus. Multiple variations on this principle exist.

Immune-Mediated Detection of Virus Protein

Common methods used in studies to detect virus infection are variations on immune-mediated methodology – using an antibody probe to bind to a viral target. Monoclonal or polyclonal antibody (discussed in Chapter 4) probes can be used. Antibody (labeled in one of many ways) that binds to virus antigen(s) will indicate the presence of the virus.[3,4]

Prior to the use of molecular nucleic acid methods to detect viruses, clinicians and investigators often used antibody-based methods. These relied on the specificity of an antibody, which was coupled with a label. The label served as a means to visualize the location of the antibody when it bound to a virus-infected cell. The presence of the label could be used to detect a virus infection (yes-no answer), including the cellular site of the virus within an infected organ. Semiquantitative results could be estimated from the intensity of the label.

The keys to immunodetection methods are the specificity of the particular antibody (the probe) used to bind to the antigen (the target). Second is the type of label attached to the antibody to identify its location.

IMMUNOHISTOCHEMISTRY

The antibody probe to be used is labeled so that it can be detected when it binds to the virus protein antigen (target), for example, in the cells of a biopsy. The cells of the biopsy would then be examined under a microscope to evaluate the localization of the labeled target. This use of labeled antibody is known as the direct method.

More commonly used is the indirect method. Here, unlabeled antibody, for example, antibody raised in a rabbit, to a virus (primary antibody) is used to bind to virus protein antigen in a biopsy. Then a second antibody is used to bind to the primary antibody. The second antibody is labeled, and the label is detected by microscopy. This use of an unlabeled primary antibody against a virus and then use of a labeled antibody to the primary antibody is termed the "indirect method."

Although requiring a second step, the indirect method has often been the preferred technique, since the labeled secondary antibody could be used in multiple studies. For example, to study various antigens, as long as rabbit antibody against each is used as the primary antibody, the same labeled secondary antibody (for example, made in a goat against rabbit antibody) could be used.

Early immunohistochemistry studies of this type utilized a fluorescent label (and fluorescence microscopy) to localize the site of binding of the primary antibody. Subsequently, other methods of labeling were developed, including peroxidase-antiperoxidase and avidin-biotin labeling. The underlying principle of these immunohistochemistry methods is the detection of antigen, such as viral protein in cells by the binding of known specific antibody.

An example of peroxidase-antiperoxidase immunohistochemistry identification of viral antigen (protein) is seen in Figure 1.1.

A variation on the immunohistochemical detection of virus is to first grow virus that might be present in cell culture, and then detect that virus by immunohistochemistry. For example, virus from a nasopharyngeal swab would be grown in cell culture. Virus that grows in the cell culture would then be definitively identified by an immunohistochemistry method as above.

For all immunohistochemical procedures, antibody specific for an virus in question must be used.

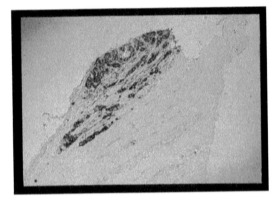

Figure 1.1 Peroxidase-antiperoxidase detection of virus. Presence of herpes simplex virus antigen in a mouse trigeminal ganglion is indicated by the dark label in multiple neurons and supporting cells. The neurons are of the first division (the ophthalmic division) of the trigeminal ganglion.

ENZYME-LINKED IMMUNOSORBENT ASSAY (ELISA)

Although more commonly used to detect and quantitate amounts of antibody, for example, antibody in the serum of patients (Chapter 4), with slight technical modifications, enzyme-linked immunosorbent assay (ELISA) testing can be used to detect antigen, such as virus.

In brief, to detect virus, known antibody to the virus would be bound to the well of a plastic plate. A liquid preparation of the unknown clinical sample to be investigated (for example, a nasopharyngeal swab in saline) would be placed on that. If specific virus is present in the throat swab sample, it will be bound to (be captured by) the specific antibody bound to the plastic plate. Then known, labeled, antibody to the virus would be added. The presence of the label of the second antibody would be evidence of the virus.

For the detection of viral antibody (Chapter 4) rather than to detect viral antigen, known viral antigen would be bound to the plastic plate.

Serum from a patient would be added, and binding of antibody (primary antibody) present in the patient's serum will occur. A secondary labeled antibody would then be used to determine the presence and the amount of the primary antibody.

LATERAL FLOW TECHNOLOGY

This immune methodology is possibly best known from its use as a pregnancy test: labeled antibody to human chorionic gonadotropin detects the presence of this hormone in the urine of pregnant women. Lateral flow technology is usually considered to give a yes-no answer. Similar methodology has been adapted to determine the presence of other antigens, with recent emphasis on the detection of SARS-CoV-2. Stability of the antibody in the kit to the virus is most important.

Lateral flow methodology can be used in home test kits to investigate nasal swabs for the presence of viral protein (antigen). Nasal swab material can be tested for SARS-CoV-2 protein (antigen), with results being provided in a very short time. Appropriate sample preparation is important, and there are likely to be more false negatives with this methodology than by other methods. On the other hand, it is very convenient.

WESTERN BLOT

After the electrophoretic separation of the viral proteins and blotting, viral antigen may be detected with labeled specific antibody to the viral antigen. Continuing with geography and building on the Southern and northern blot terminology, when antibody is used to detect antigen in a blot after gel electrophoresis, the technique has often been termed a western blot study. Probe antibody may be polyclonal or monoclonal. As above, a primary antibody is typically used to bind to the target antigen or antigens, and a labeled secondary antibody used to bind to the first antibody.

NOMENCLATURE OF BLOT STUDIES

As noted above, the procedure by which target DNA fragments are separated by gel electrophoresis and after transfer to a blot are detected by use of labeled DNA probes was developed by Edwin Southern. The procedure, therefore, has often been termed a Southern blot study. Shortly thereafter, a similar procedure was used to separate RNA fragments which after blotting were probed with labeled DNA probes. With slight tongue in cheek, this procedure was termed a northern blot study. Subsequently, protein studies were termed western blots. And there are southwestern blots (DNA-protein) and northeastern blots (RNA-protein).

VISUALIZATION OF VIRUS BY ELECTRON MICROSCOPY

Although viruses are very small, they can be seen by electron microscopy. Viruses are usually measured in terms of nanometers.

  1 inch = 2.54 centimeters (cm)
  1 cm = 10 millimeters (mm)
  1mm = 1,000 micrometers (µm)
  1 µm = 1,000 nanometers (nm)
Therefore, 1 inch = 25,400,000 nm

The size of poliomyelitis virus is about 30 (~30) nm, human herpes simplex virus is ~150 nm, and SARS-CoV-2 is ~130 nm. For comparison, a red blood cell is ~8 µm (8,000 nm). The largest human virus is the smallpox virus, which is ~400 nm. Some giant viruses have been reported, up to 1,500 nm in size. However, there is no evidence that such giant virus, sometimes termed "girus," infects humans.

A single virus particle is often referred to as a virion. The term does not indicate whether the particle is infectious or not. Polyoma virus particles seen by electron microscopy the brain of a patient with progressive multifocal leukoencephalopathy (PML) are shown in Figure 6.1 in Chapter 6.

VIRUS CAN BE GROWN AND QUANTITATED IN CELL CULTURE: THE PLAQUE ASSAY

Other than by the growth of infectious virus in cell culture, the above methods do not definitively indicate the presence of infectious virus. Methods to measure amounts of infectious virus are discussed in Chapter 2.

With all methods the problems of false negatives (virus is there but goes undetected) need be considered. False positives (virus is not there but the test reads out that it is) is usually a lesser problem.

Antibody to Viruses

Viral proteins have often been discussed as their being viral antigens. Such antigens often lead to the production of antibody by individuals infected with the virus. Antibodies are made by infected individuals as a reaction by their protective immune systems. These antibodies are present in convalescent immune serum (or plasma) of people after they recover from infection or after immunization with a vaccine.[5]

When multiple immune cells in humans respond to an infection or to vaccine immunization by making antibody, they make polyclonal antibody. The viral proteins to which the immune cells respond are complex (for example, SARS-CoV-2 spikes), and so the parts of the spike to which one immune cell responds may be different from another, even if they are both responding to the viral spike. The specific part of the spike protein to which an immune cell responds is termed the "epitope."

Each of the many immune cells that respond to an infection makes a single type of antibody to the epitope it recognized. Therefore, convalescent immune blood would be expected to contain multiple antibodies made by multiple immune cells (polyclonal antibody). In the laboratory, antibody from a clone of a single cell can be developed, termed "monoclonal antibody."

When antibody is therapeutically administered to patients (termed "passive immunization"), antibody is not expected to persist in the individual. Long-term antibody, however, will persist after recovery from infection or after vaccine immunization (termed "active immunization").

The immune system is discussed further in Chapter 4.

Antiviral Medications

In addition to the use of antibody to inhibit viral infections, antiviral medications have been considered. As noted above, it has been difficult to develop antiviral medications because viruses grow only within living cells, and inhibiting viruses at those sites might also damage the cell.

Several ant-viral medications in the category of nucleoside analogs have been investigated, including remdesivir, molnupiravir, and nirmatrelvir, which are being tested in the treatment of SARS-CoV-2 infections. Antiviral medications and nucleoside analogs are discussed further in Chapters 3 and 8.

The History of Virology

With the foregoing background, the history of virology can be considered. It might date to the third century BC, based on smallpox-like lesions (rash) on the face of several Egyptian mummies. And the atrophic leg of a figure on an Egyptian stele from as early as 1500 BC has been thought to indicate poliomyelitis virus infection. Of course, at those times and for many, many years, there was no concept of viruses (or bacteria) as causes of disease. The concept of the germ (bacterial) theory of disease did not develop until the third quarter of the nineteenth century through the work of Louis Pasteur and Edward Koch. Consideration of disease causation by particles smaller than bacteria did not develop until later, through the work of Dmitri Ivanovsky and Martinus Beijerinck. The latter is credited with coining the word "virus." Carlos Finlay and Walter Reed described the first human virus infection, yellow fever, in 1900 (Chapter 7).

Several recent pandemics have been caused by viruses, including AIDS caused by HIV.

Subsequent to the widespread influenza virus pandemic of 1918–1919, the largest influenza virus pandemics were those of 1957–1958 (Asian flu) and 1968–1969 (Hong Kong flu). The COVID-19 pandemic caused by a novel coronavirus, probably bat-related (discussed below), has been very much in recent news.

The first well-described viral pandemic was the influenza pandemic of 1918–1919. As is the case with many respiratory illnesses, infections likely started as an infection of the upper respiratory tract and in more severe cases included the lower respiratory tract. The upper respiratory tract includes the nose, pharynx, and larynx, and the lower respiratory tract includes the lungs. That pandemic has been estimated to have killed more than 50 million people, possibly ~5% of the population of the world. Many people probably died of bacterial infection superimposed on the viral infection. Antibiotics, to say nothing of antiviral medications, were not available.

In the COVID-19 pandemic, ~0.05% of the population of the world is thought to have died.

For a historical comparison, the Black Death in 1348–1352, caused by the bacterium *Yersinia pestis*, killed ~50% of the population of Europe.

Influenza virus is a single-stranded RNA virus. Influenza types A, B, and C infect humans, with the great majority being due to influenza type

A. Vaccines exist, but the virus often changes slightly year to year, which may decrease the effectiveness of any one vaccine.[6]

In discussing the SARS-CoV-2, the cause of the COVID-19 pandemic, it was noted previously that protein spikes are present on the outside of each virion (virus particle). For influenza virus, proteins are also on the surface of the virus particles, and these have been well characterized. The two primary influenza virus proteins, which are targets of influenza vaccines, are the neuraminidase (N) and the hemagglutinin (H). Since these virus proteins often change over time, they receive numbers in accord with the change. For example, influenza A may be described as being H_1N_1 or H_7N_9. Vaccines are changed to keep in step with changes in the virus.

The 1918 influenza pandemic was caused by influenza A virus (H_1N_1), the 1957 influenza pandemic by influenza A (H_2N_2), the 1968 influenza pandemic by influenza A (H_3N_2), and the 2009 influenza pandemic by influenza A (H_1N_1).

Human coronavirus epidemics include the severe acute respiratory syndrome (SARS) in 2002–2003 and the Middle East respiratory syndrome (MERS) in 2012. The coronaviruses that caused SARS, MERS, and COVID-19, along with two other human coronaviruses that cause the common cold are members of the *Betacoronavirus* genus.

Epidemics are less widespread than are pandemics.

The HIV pandemic, starting in ~1980, continues as a worldwide problem. Other viral outbreaks in recent years have included those due to Ebola virus, Lassa fever virus, several arboviruses (dengue virus, Zika virus, yellow fever virus, West Nile virus, and chikungunya virus), and measles virus (discussed in Chapters 6 and 7).

Vaccines have been developed to treat (to prevent) viral and other infections. The history of vaccines may start with the smallpox virus vaccine of Edward Jenner (1796) and the rabies virus vaccine of Louis Pasteur (1885). Vaccines are further discussed in Chapter 4.

Antigenic Shift and Antigenic Drift

Many viruses, particularly some RNA viruses, show major (antigenic shift) or minor (antigenic drift) changes year to year. As discussed in Chapter 3, mutations occur spontaneously due to nucleic acid (DNA or RNA) changes. Those that are deleterious to the replication of the virus will obviously not be passed on to new virus. Those that increase viral infectivity or rate of virus replication may lead to increased infection. However, there is complexity in that increased infection in one animal host may not have the same effect in another animal host, and an altered virus may enhance immune responsiveness of the infected individual.

Influenza A may change its H and N and be resistant to antibodies that had been raised against its prior H and N forms. The changes are random and are manifest when the changes happen to enhance viral infectivity or replication. Subsequently, these viral advantages may be lost as the host adapts. For some RNA viruses such as influenza, such viral changes may be a clinical problem. Fortunately, measles virus, which like influenza virus is also a single-stranded RNA virus and which in the past often caused severe illness, does not appear to make these changes.

The year-to-year variation of influenza virus, in which there may be clinical significance in the changes, is more the exception than the rule among viruses. Emphasized is that virus variants occur during infections by random changes in the RNA or DNA genome of the viruses. Viral variants are common, although such variations are more common with RNA than with DNA viruses.[7]

Multiple variants have been described for SARS-CoV-2, with reports noting that one variant or another may be more infectious or more pathogenic. Emphasized has been whether variants are inhibited by currently available vaccines.

In considering yearly influenza, the usual question is whether the influenza virus of the year is susceptible to the vaccine previously administered. The jury is still out on the clinical importance of SARS-CoV-2 variants, and a conservative viewpoint is probably most reasonable. The clinical importance of some variants and their control with present vaccines is not yet clearly known.[8,9]

At the time of writing this book, more than 15 SARS-CoV-2 variants and subvariants have been described, most recently BA.5.

As discussed in Chapter 4, vaccines against SARS-CoV-2 virus emphasize immune reactivity to the surface "spikes" of the virus. Unless those change, similar to the changes that occur in the hemagglutinin (H) and neuraminidase (N) of influenza virus, vaccines are likely to be effective against SARS-CoV-2 variants. Since different RNA and non-RNA vaccines focus on different antigens, some have said it may make sense for "booster" shots in the future to be of vaccines other than the vaccine the individual initially received.

Evolution of Viruses

Before discussing the evolution of viruses, brief mention will be made of the possible effects of viruses on evolution. One could speculate on dinosaur viruses and viruses of other extinct animals and hypothesize a possible viral role in extinctions.

Somewhat less speculatively are endogenous retroviral elements (DNA copies of RNA viruses) that are present in animal cells, including humans. They are further discussed in Chapter 6. These elements likely were important in the evolution of cells, and one may consider their possible role in human evolution. These elements exist at present as parts of human cells and play a role in cellular functions. Some have speculated on their being responsible for some human illnesses.

Since viruses can only live (replicate) in living cells, some have reasonably thought that although they seem very primitive, they must have developed after living cells developed. Possibly they developed as pieces of the RNA of bacteria or other early organisms. It is generally thought that early life was RNA based, and only later in evolution did the DNA basis that we know today develop.

Because viruses are either RNA or DNA, if viruses developed from primitive organisms, it might suggest two such events, one for RNA viruses (developing from RNA-based organisms) and later one for DNA viruses (developing from DNA-based organisms). That might then require concluding that the panoply of currently existing RNA viruses developed from some primordial RNA virus, and DNA viruses from some similar early DNA virus. Alternatively, there may have been multiple virus from RNA events and also virus from DNA events. Lastly, it is interesting to speculate on the possibility that present DNA viruses evolved from a primordial RNA virus.

Clearer than this speculation is the likelihood that some viruses of animals have evolved to infect humans. An example of this is the likelihood that measles virus developed from rinderpest virus, a virus of cattle. It is thought that measles virus developed ~1,000 to 500 BC in conjunction with cattle farming. In the instance of rinderpest, it is likely a new virus developed, that measles virus developed from rinderpest virus. It is not thought that humans are infected with a variant of rinderpest but rather a new virus, measles virus. Interestingly, rinderpest is currently thought to have been eliminated from cattle. Measles virus is also closely related to canine distemper virus.

An interesting area of speculation might be the time of origin of smallpox virus, which probably developed from a rodent pox virus. When Europeans first came to America, there was devastating loss of life from smallpox, suggesting that Native Americans had very little resistance to the virus. While not at all immune to the virus, Europeans had more resistance than did Native Americans. Second, America was populated by travelers coming across the Behring Strait about 20,000 years ago. Together, these observations might be taken to hypothesize that smallpox virus developed in Europe/Asia/Africa less than 20,000 years ago.

In other instances, rather than the evolution of new human viruses, viruses of animals have on occasion infected humans, and this occurs at the present. For example, avian influenza and swine influenza virus may infect humans. Such viruses have a mixture of human influenza and swine or avian influenza genes. One could argue whether such a virus is variant of an animal virus or is a new virus. Random mutations in influenza virus that increase infections, for example, in avian hosts, may not increase infections in humans.

Several viral zoonoses, viral infections of animals that are transmitted to humans, are discussed in Chapter 6.

Changes in viruses to facilitate viral infection of cells not previously infectable by the virus may occur by spontaneous mutation of specific viral genes and by recombination. As noted below, in discussing the origins of SARS-CoV-2, this gain of function is sometimes enhanced in the study of viruses. Viral recombinants may also occur spontaneously during infection. In recombination events, the genes of a virus are mixed with the genes of another virus and a novel, "hybrid" virus is produced.[10,11]

Lastly, it is noted that viruses have been synthesized from "off the shelf" chemicals, the best example of this being poliomyelitis virus.[12]

Poliomyelitis virus is an RNA virus. Since the entire sequence of the viral RNA genome was known, adding RNA nucleotides to a framework until the entire RNA sequence was constructed was possible. Infectious poliomyelitis virus was thus made de novo. The argument in favor of this process is that greater understanding of viral functions will be obtained. Philosophically, this might lend support to the conclusion that viruses are not alive. Ethically, one could question the de novo construction of infectious virus on safety grounds.

Origin of SARS-CoV-2 Virus

Where did the SARS-CoV-2 virus come from? The answer of course is not definitively known.[13,14] What appears to be true is that the first infections appeared in Wuhan, China. Second, the Wuhan Institute of Virology was probably the most active coronavirus laboratory in the world, and it had stored many bat coronavirus isolates. Third, coronavirus isolated from an individual in Wuhan in December 2019 had more than 96% similarity with a bat coronavirus from a cave in China.

Important is that it has not been difficult to adapt coronaviruses to grow in human cells, done in order to more fully study them.[13] This is sometimes termed "gain of function."

The above is circumstantial evidence relative to the COVID-19 pandemic. A reasonable hypothesis is that bat coronavirus was altered so that it grew well in human cells in order to be more completely studied. The virus then escaped from the Wuhan laboratory by accidentally infecting laboratory personnel, who then accidentally infected others in Wuhan.

Epidemiology

Given the importance and recent emphasis on epidemiology in considering viral infections, a brief discussion of some aspects of epidemiology follows.

In the recent past, epidemiology was emphasized in considerations of viral infections and autoimmune illnesses of the nervous system, including influenza virus vaccine as a cause of Guillain-Barré syndrome, West Nile virus of meningitis/encephalitis, and Zika virus infection as a cause of microcephaly.

More recently, epidemiology has been brought to the forefront in considerations of COVID-19. For example, PCR testing of nasopharyngeal swabs for SARS-CoV-2 RNA in asymptomatic individuals is primarily an epidemiological issue. The primary goal in these studies is not to care for and treat the individuals (they are asymptomatic) but to follow and alter the transmission of SARS-CoV-2 infection in the population.

While the goals of epidemiology and of clinical medicine are largely the same, to minimize human illnesses, including viral infections, their means and points of emphasis sometimes differ and are interesting to consider.[15]

In very brief, epidemiology emphasizes groups of people, and clinical medicine emphasizes individuals. Of course, if treatment is found to be effective in epidemiological studies of groups of individuals, that would be very important for individuals. Similarly, insights gained from evaluating individual patients may lead to formulating epidemiological studies.

In many ways, these approaches are complementary. Epidemiological studies noted the importance of blood pressure control in populations of people to decrease stroke and heart disease. At present, when a patient sees a clinical medicine physician, blood pressure measurement and means to control blood pressure are greatly emphasized. Epidemiological studies also noted the relationship between smoking and lung cancer, and this is currently a major point of emphasis in clinical medicine.

Preludes to these epidemiological studies were the clinical observations that elevated blood pressure seemed important as a cause of stroke and heart disease. And initial clinical observations that there seemed to be a relationship between cigarette smoking and lung cancer led to epidemiological studies to investigate the relationship.

Early clinical observations of the COVID-19 pandemic suggested the importance of age on survival, and this has been important in epidemiological investigations. However, even if one discusses differences based on age, it would remain necessary to determine what about age is important. Impaired immune responsiveness of the very young and the very old is often cited when considering infectious illnesses.[16,17]

Several of the many points important in considerations of epidemiology are briefly discussed here.

PROBABILITY AND STATISTICS

How would one investigate the importance of age, of pregnancy, or of ethnicity and COVID-19? A general start might be to compare groups of people, to determine whether people with the trait being studied differ in illness severity than do others. The goal would be to determine the probability that that the trait is important in illness progression.

Many studies in the past emphasized the probability (the p) that smoking caused lung cancer. Others have investigated the p of an antiviral medication curing a patient with an illness. The P is a means to predict the future, albeit not with 100% accuracy.

Common to both epidemiology and clinical medicine is the use of statistics to estimate the P, the likelihood that smoking will cause lung cancer in an individual, and the likelihood that the antiviral medication will cure the patient. The accurate determination of the P is the quest, but because of the many variables in determining disease occurrence, severity and cure, statistics need be used.

A significant P, indicating benefit of a medication may be thought of as follows. If a medication is more than 1,000-fold more likely to produce a beneficial effect than is no treatment (or treatment with a placebo), the P is significant.

So, $P < .001$ indicates the likelihood, the probability of a beneficial effect occurring simply by chance is less than 1 in 1,000. If on testing the medication, the $P < .001$ it would be reasonable to conclude that the beneficial effect (B) after treatment (T) is not simply due to chance.

Almost any treatment may seem to be effective, because some people will do well with no treatment. If 10 people out of 100 do well with no treatment, how many out of 100 would need to do well to demonstrate the benefit of a particular treatment? Appropriate statistical methods may provide the answer.

PLACEBO AND NOCEBO EFFECTS

Many issues come up in treatment studies, and statistics may be useful in attempting to determine the *P*. Placebo and nocebo occurrences are two.

Efficacy of treatment is most easily determined in double-blinded, placebo-controlled trials. In determining the *P* of medication efficacy, such trials are the gold standard. When neither the patient nor the treating physician knows whether the patient has received the medication being tested (active medication) or a placebo ("sugar pill"), efficacy may most clearly be determined.

Interestingly, in many studies, the symptoms of some patients receiving the placebo improve – termed the "placebo effect" This is particularly an issue in testing medications to treat pain, where improvement with the placebo may occur in about 30% of treated individuals. Many are aware of reports of individuals who were injured but did not report pain – because of circumstances at the time. This may be thought of as an effect of the mind. The placebo effect may be related to such a mind effect. In testing the efficacy of a medication, the P of improvement need be significantly greater than that of the placebo.

The nocebo effect is the flip side of the placebo effect, and in some ways, it is even more interesting, in terms of a mind effect. In trials where a beneficial placebo effect may be noted in some, others may develop adverse side effects to the placebo, the sugar pill, termed the "nocebo effect."[18] Since the administration of all medications is predicated on a risk:benefit ratio, nocebo-related side effects (risks) may have an effect on whether a medication is used.

Typically, placebo and nocebo effects are thought to be related to information given to patients at the time of clinical trials. Patients in trials are informed as to the possible benefits of the medication being tested (including the improvement of symptoms) and potential adverse side effects of the medication being tested. In such trials, patients do not know whether they received the active medication being tested or the placebo, but patients usually believe that they received the active medication.

PCR TESTING OF ASYMPTOMATIC PEOPLE

In the past, clinicians would likely have performed PCR testing to determine the possible presence of an infectious agent in patients with suggestive symptoms. If the patient did not have symptoms such as fever, congestion, cough, shortness of breath, headache, such PCR testing would likely not have been performed – in the pre–COVID-19 world. This has changed with COVID-19, in large part by epidemiological concerns of the spread of infection.

In terms of screening for SARS-CoV-2 virus, epidemiologists emphasized PCR testing of nasopharyngeal swabs in large numbers of people, including people without clinical symptoms of illness. Goals included understanding how the virus spreads among people and plans to isolate virus-positive people from others to limit disease transmission.

However, the data has also led to an interesting conclusion that may have widespread future impact. As discussed above, SARS-CoV-2, PCR-positive individuals have often been considered as being cases of COVID-19, including individuals who were asymptomatic. Should individuals who are SARS-CoV-2, PCR-positive but who are asymptomatic be considered as COVID-19 cases? Possibly not.

However, it is not so simple. It is well known that people shed various types of viruses and may be asymptomatic. Some are treated for the asymptomatic infection. If they are treated, should they not be thought of as cases of infection?

For example, people with asymptomatic genital herpes simplex virus (HSV) infection may be treated with medications such as acyclovir (Chapters 5 and 8). The medications do not eliminate their infections, and they are treated primarily to prevent their transmitting the virus to others – an epidemiological concern. They may be considered as cases of HSV infection, even though they are asymptomatic.

All people who shed virus, including those that are asymptomatic, may be thought of as having at least a low-level virus infection. Virus is being produced in infected cells, and probably those cells are being destroyed – lytic infection is present (Chapter 5). Treatment of virus-positive but asymptomatic individuals will likely receive much future discussion. This blurs the distinction between epidemiology and clinical medicine.

Therapeutic Viruses and Atypical Agents

This introductory virology chapter will close with an introduction of unusual viruses and virus-like atypical agents.

VIRUS VECTORS

Some viruses have been used as a means to treat human genetic illnesses. Such viruses have been modified to incorporate specific human DNA genes and are then used as vectors to bring this DNA into human cells. These viruses are also modified to decrease their disease-causing capability. Virus vectors are further discussed in Chapters 3 and 9.

BACTERIOPHAGE

Interestingly, some viruses can infect, reproduce in, and thereby kill bacteria. Such virus, termed "bacteriophage" (or "phage"), has been considered as possible treatment for some bacterial infections. A specific type of bacteriophage would need be used to treat a specific bacterial infection. It would be important to use selective bacteriophage, so that "good" bacteria are not destroyed. The same selective concept is considered in the development of antibiotics. Bacteriophage therapy has taken a back seat to antibiotic use in treating human bacterial infections, but it may be of real value in the future; viruses may be used to control animal and plant pathogens.[19] For example, AgriPhage is a bacteriophage approved for agricultural use in the United States.

It should also be noted, however, that bacteriophages may have deleterious effects. Specific bacteriophages that infect diphtheria and cholera bacteria may lead to those bacteria producing toxins that are the mark of clinical diphtheria and cholera. Specific bacteriophage contribute the genes for those toxins, without which the bacteria do not produce the toxins.

ONCOLYTIC VIRUSES

Viruses have also been considered as possible therapeutic agents in the treatment of cancer. Varied types of such oncolytic viruses have been studied. A type of herpes simplex virus mutant termed "thymidine kinase negative" (TK neg.) is one such viral mutant that has been studied. This viral mutant grows well in dividing cells (presumably by using the high levels of nucleosides and cellular replication enzymes that are present in these types of cells) but not in nondividing cells (which have low levels of nucleosides and replication enzymes). Some investigators have studied TK neg. mutants for their potential in treating cancer, where rapidly dividing cells are present.

Since neurons (nerve cells) are nondividing cells, TK neg. mutants of this type have also been used to investigate infections of neurons (Chapter 8). The use of oncolytic viruses is further discussed in Chapter 9.

ATYPICAL AGENTS

While the emphasis of this volume is on viruses and viral illnesses, discussion of atypical "virus-like" agents is included. Among these unusual agents are endogenous retroviral elements, virusoids, viroids, and prions. The importance of these agents relates in part not only to illnesses they may cause but also to human biology and speculatively to evolution. At the beginning of this chapter, the question was raised as to definitions of living organisms and whether viruses were living organisms. If it can be questioned as to what type of organism viruses are, the difficulty in categorizing the atypical agents is even more difficult.

Endogenous retroviral elements are RNA retroviruses, which as DNA proviruses have become part of the DNA of cells, including human cells (introduced above, in the section Evolution of Viruses). Their functions are part of human biology and biochemistry. It is possibly reasonable to conclude that while their incorporation in cells was a type of infection in the very distant past, at present any disease related to them is more in the category of a metabolic illness than infection.

Mitochondria, another type of endogenous element, is discussed in Chapter 3.

Virusoids are pieces of RNA that cannot replicate, unless they receive biochemical aid from viruses which coinfect cells with the virusoids. And viroids are even more primitive, and they require biochemical aid from the cells that they infect (Chapter 6). Are these primitive entities from which viruses evolved, or did they develop subsequent to the development of viruses and cells, upon which they are dependent for replication?[20]

Lastly are prions, "infectious" proteins that contain neither RNA nor DNA. Amazingly, prion diseases can not only be inherited (genetically transmitted) but are also infectious, and "replicate" by causing normal protein to become abnormal (Chapter 7).[21]

The Future of Virology

Important for the future of clinical virology are the new mRNA techniques to develop vaccines. The use of RNA techniques to develop vaccines (discussed in Chapter 4) will hopefully keep pace with any new viruses that appear. RNA vaccines may also be of use in bacterial and in other infections. Might they also be useful in the treatment of cancer?

Also, the great progress in antibiotic development in the last quarter of the twentieth century may well be followed by similar progress in antiviral medication development. The development of effective antivirals, probably first dating from the development of acyclovir (Chapter 8) and given a big boost by the development of antivirals to treat HIV (Chapter 3), will very likely grow as the result of COVID-19. Remdesivir, molnupiravir, ritonavir, and nirmatrelvir are among the antivirals being tested in the treatment of SARS-CoV-2 infections (Chapter 3).

The future of virology is more thoroughly considered in Chapter 9.

Next, Chapter 2 returns to more traditional virology, with emphasis on the means to measure infectious virus particles by the viral plaque assay.

Further Reading

MJ Hewlett, D Camerini, DC Bloom. *Basic Virology*, 4th ed., Wiley Blackwell, 2022

J Louten. *Essential Human Virology*, Elsevier, 2016

MD Waters, A Dhawan, T Marrs, et al. *The Coronavirus Pandemic and the Future.* Vol. 2: *Virology, Epidemiology, Translational Toxicology and Therapeutics,* Royal Society of Chemistry, 2022

MR Wilson, KL Tyler. The current status of next-generation sequencing for diagnosis of central nervous system infections. *JAMA Neurol* 2022;**79**:**1095–1096**. https://doi.org/10.1001/jamaneurol.2002.2287

E Cahan. As superbugs flourish, bacteriophage therapy recaptures researchers' interest. JAMA 2023;329:781–784. https://doi.org/jama.2022.17756

Measurement of Infectious Virus

The Measurement of Virus Plaque-Forming Units (PFUs), Where Each PFU Represents an Infectious Virus Particle

Discussion in this chapter presents methods to directly measure the number of infectious virus particles in a sample. Methods to directly inhibit the infectivity of virus particles in a sample by antibody are then presented – the measurement of neutralizing antibody.

As noted in Chapter 1, multiple methods are available to count or quantitate the amount of virus present in a sample. For example, this may be done by directly counting the number of viral particles seen by electron microscopy – if 1,000 viral particles are seen in 1/1,000 of a sample (very small amounts can be studied at one time by electron microscopy), it would be concluded that 1,000,000 virus particles were present in the initial sample.

Alternatively, biochemical methods may be used, such as the measurement of viral RNA in a sample. Since each SARS-CoV-2 virus particle contains a specific amount of RNA, if the amount of viral RNA in a sample is equal to 1,000,000 times that amount, it would be concluded that 1,000,000 virus particles were present.

These and some other methods suffer from the drawback that they do not measure amounts of infectious virus present. The electron microscopic evaluation would observe physical virus particles that are infectious and those that are not. The biochemical method would measure viral RNA, including from noninfectious particles and disrupted, "broken" particles. To measure the amount of infectious virus present in a sample, use of an assay that includes virus particle infectivity need be used – the plaque assay.[22]

Viruses can only infect, grow, and reproduce in living cells. Therefore, to count numbers of infectious virus particles, the assay need be performed in living cells. As noted in Chapter 1, different viruses infect different types of cells from different animal species (including humans). For that reason, it is necessary to select appropriate cell types when doing plaque assays. The example described below is typical of a plaque assay for herpes simplex virus (HSV), as performed in the author's laboratory.

HSV commonly causes "cold sores" on the face as well as genital area infections. As discussed in Chapter 5, HSV frequently establishes latent infections in nerve cells (neurons), and with reactivation of latent infections, recurrent facial, eye, or genital infection occurs. HSV may also cause a brain infection, HSV encephalitis (Chapter 6).

CELL CULTURE

Cells in which to grow viruses are usually cell lines or primary cells. Cell lines are commonly used, since they can be grown and divided and grown and divided many times. Cell lines can be obtained from cancer or noncancer tissues. A monkey cell line (Vero cells) has been commonly used to grow HSV, as are HeLa cells, a cell line developed from the cervical cancer of a woman named Henrietta Lacks.

Alternatively, primary cells can be used. Primary cells are directly obtained from animal or human sources and can be grown and divided only a few times. An interesting human primary cell type is human foreskin epithelial cells, obtained after circumcision. In some instances, primary cells maintain characteristics of the tissues from which they were obtained – investigators may study the functions of neurons in cell culture and the contractions of muscle cells.

Herpes simplex virus grows in several types of cell lines and primary cells, more so than a number of other viruses.

After the dispersion of cells into suspensions of individual cells (from stocks stored in a freezer, cell lines, or cells from tissue, primary cells), accomplished with enzymes such as trypsin, the cells are grown in plates in cell culture.

Cells are grown as monolayers, sheets of cells one cell thick. They are typically grown in sterile plastic plates, covered with liquid growth medium (electrolyte-balanced and containing growth factors and glucose) and are incubated at body temperature (37°C). Antibiotics are included in the culture medium to prevent bacterial growth. Cells settle on the plastic plates and grow and divide until the entire surface of the plate is covered by the cell monolayer.

When microscopic examination shows that the monolayer has covered the complete surface of the plastic plate, it is possible to perform a plaque assay to determine the number of infectious virus particles in a sample.

PERFORMANCE OF THE PLAQUE ASSAY

The sample to be evaluated for number of infectious virus particles is placed in sterile cell culture medium or saline. For example, a saline-moistened swab of a human skin lesion might be placed in a tube containing saline and the number of infectious virus particles determined; virus so directly isolated from a patient is seen in Figure 8.1 in Chapter 8.

Alternatively, as in a laboratory example to follow, virus is first grown in cell culture, and the number of infectious particles in that virus-infected culture then determined.

Viruses can reproduce enormously, and so if medium containing virus grown in culture is directly placed on monolayers for a plaque assay, the entire monolayer very likely would be destroyed by the large number of infectious virus particles present. Quantitation (counting of individual plaques) then would not be possible. Serial dilution of the specimen to be tested avoids this problem. An example of appropriate serial dilution methodology to determine the number of infectious HSV particles is as follows.

From culture fluid containing HSV to be quantitated (Tube XX), 0.1 ml is removed and placed into a tube containing 0.9 ml of sterile medium (Tube #1). The original culture fluid has, therefore, been diluted 10-fold (a 1:10 dilution).

From Tube #1, 0.1 ml is removed under sterile conditions and placed in 0.9 ml of fresh, sterile cell culture medium (Tube #2). The original 0.1 ml of virus-containing medium (Tube XX) has, therefore, been diluted 100-fold (1:100).

Further, 10-fold dilutions are made based on an estimate of how many infectious HSV particles might be present. Estimates as varied as 10 to 1,000,000 infectious particles per 0.1 ml might be considered.

For example, 10-fold dilutions of the original culture fluid (Tube XX) might be carried out 5 times.

Tube #1 – 0.1 ml of original XX culture fluid is put in a tube containing 0.9 ml of sterile culture fluid.

Therefore, original XX fluid has been diluted 10-fold, a 1:10 dilution.

Tube #2 – 0.1 ml from Tube #1 is put into 0.9 ml of sterile culture fluid. Therefore, a 1:100 dilution.

Tube #3 – 0.1 ml from Tube #2 is put into 0.9 ml of sterile culture fluid. Therefore, a 1:1,000 dilution.

Tube #4 – 0.1 ml from Tube #3 is put into 0.9 ml of sterile culture fluid. Therefore, a 1:10,000 dilution.

Tube #5 – 0.1 ml from Tube #4 is put into 0.9 ml of sterile culture fluid. Therefore, a 1:100,000 dilution.

At this point, monolayer plates are prepared for testing. The culture medium in each plate overlying the cell monolayer is discarded. Each tube of virus-containing fluid (Tubes #1–#5) is tested in duplicate, two monolayer plates for each tube.

From Tube #1, 0.1 ml is dropped onto each of two monolayer plates. Two monolayer plates are similarly infected for each of Tubes #2, #3, #4, and #5. All 10 plates are then incubated at 37°C for 1 hour. They are then removed from the incubator, cell culture medium added, and the plates further incubated at 37°C for several days. This last incubation period varies among viruses, based on the expected growth rate of different viruses. For HSV, this is usually 4 days. After 4 days, the medium is removed. Monolayers are then "fixed" (fluid added to kill the monolayer cells and any virus present), stained, and dried. At that point, "plaques" in each plate are counted.

Each plaque is an area of cells destroyed by the virus (plaques do not stain) and easily visualized against the background of stained intact monolayer cells. The key premise of the plaque assay is that each infectious virus particle in the fluid being tested (Tubes #1–#5) will infect one monolayer cell. Each infected monolayer cell results in virus being reproduced, which infects adjacent cells. This cycle is repeated multiple times, resulting in an area of dead cells – the plaque.

Each plaque indicates one infectious virus particle, a plaque-forming unit (PFU).

Interpretation of the Plaque Assay

Fluid from Tubes #1 and #2 might contain so much virus that it destroys the whole monolayer, and it is impossible to count individual plaques. In each of the two plates tested with fluid from Tube #3, there may be more than 100 plaques, and it is difficult to make an accurate count. It might be impossible to differentiate one plaque from another.

In plates infected with fluid from Tube #4, plaques are readily counted, for example, 22 in one plate and 14 in the other – an average of 18 plaques per plate. In plates infected with fluid from Tube #5, one plate has 2 plaques and the other 0 plaques. In this example, data from plates infected with fluid from Tube #4 would be used. The process is summarized in Table 2.1.

Table 2.1 **Determination of viral plaque-forming units (PFUs)**			
Tube #	**Volume removed and put into 0.9 ml medium in the next tube**	**Dilution of the original virus-infected fluid**	**0.1 ml from each tube cultured on each of 2 plates, number of viral PFUs per plate**
Tube XX of virus-containing fluid to be tested	0.1 ml	None	ND
#1	0.1 ml	10-fold	Too numerous to count in both plates
#2	0.1 ml	100-fold	Too numerous to count in both plates
#3	0.1 ml	1,000-fold	More than 100 in both plates
#4	0.1 ml	10,000-fold	20/16; average of 18 plaques
#5	ND	100,000-fold	0/2

ND = not done.

There was an average of 18 plaques per plate, from the two plates each infected with 0.1 ml from Tube #4. Since Tube #4 had been diluted 10,000-fold (relative to the original XX culture fluid), it would be concluded that original XX culture fluid contained 180,000 ($18 \times 10,000$) infectious HSV particles per each 0.1 ml, written in exponential form as 1.8×10^5 PFUs/0.1 ml.

Each of the 180,000 plaques in the 0.1 ml example represents an infectious HSV particle, a plaque-forming unit, a PFU. The assay does not say anything about noninfectious virus particles being present, which may be important in some clinical situations, such as in vaccines. Figure 8.1 in Chapter 8 is an example of an HSV plaque assay.

All testing is performed under sterile conditions. At the completion of the testing, all plasticware that contained cells or virus is autoclaved (sterilized) before being discarded.

Plaque assays to detect infectious SARS-CoV-2 could be performed using nasopharyngeal swabs from individuals or swabs of hard surfaces, but it would be a much more time-consuming process than is rapid polymerase chain reaction (PCR) testing to detect viral RNA. To return to reports that SARS-CoV-2 virus can "live" on hard surfaces: if SARS-CoV-2 in a swab from a hard surface (for example, a park bench) was detected in a plaque assay, it would be evidence that infectious virus was present.

Renato Dulbecco won the Nobel Prize in Physiology/Medicine in 1975, in part for developing the viral plaque assay.

MEASUREMENT OF VIRUS NEUTRALIZING ANTIBODY BY PLAQUE ASSAY: PLAQUE REDUCTION METHOD

Another use of the plaque assay is the measurement of neutralizing antibody, antibody that blocks virus infectivity. Antibody production, including neutralizing antibody after a viral infection or after receiving a vaccine, is discussed in Chapter 4.

At this point, discussion now focuses on how neutralizing antibody may be biologically measured by the inhibition of the infectivity of known virus. Neutralizing antibody blocks virus from infecting cells – it neutralizes it.

If a known amount of infectious virus (a known number of viral PFUs) is incubated with human serum containing antibody to the virus, the expected number of PFUs in a subsequent plaque assay will be decreased. The decrease in PFUs will be in proportion to the amount of neutralizing antibody in the serum being tested. The neutralizing antibody titer will be determined.

The test is performed with multiple tubes, each containing a known amount of infectious virus (a known number of PFUs), and each also containing serum to be tested for neutralizing antibody. While the number of viral PFUs in each tube is constant, the serum to be tested is serially diluted.

For example, stock virus known to contain 100 PFUs of SARS-CoV-2 per 0.1 ml might be used. In each of five tubes, 500 PFUs (that is, 0.5 ml) would be placed. To each tube containing 500 viral PFUs, serum from a patient's blood would be added. However, before being added to the 500 viral PFUs in each tube, the serum to be tested would be diluted.

For example, 4-fold dilutions of serum might be used, such as 1:4, 1:16, 1:64, 1:256, 1:1,024.

Determination of the number of PFUs per 0.1 ml of the virus–antibody mixture would then be performed – as for the previous plaque assay. If fewer than the expected number of plaques per 0.1 ml is seen on the plaque assay, it would be concluded that neutralizing antibody was present in the serum.

In this example, each tube contains 0.5 ml of virus suspension (total of 500 PFUs) and 0.5 ml of diluted serum (the total volume per tube is 1.0 ml). From each tube, 0.1 ml samples are tested in duplicate in a plaque assay as previously to determine the number of viral PFUs.

If there is no neutralizing antibody to the virus being tested present in the serum, it would be expected that in a plaque assay there would be ~50 PFUs per 0.1 ml. Since each tube initially contained 100 PFUs per 0.1 ml and each was diluted 1:2 (50%) by the volume of diluted serum added, 50 PFUs per 0.1 ml would be expected if no neutralizing antibody was present.

Detection of less than 50 PFUs per 0.1 ml would indicate the presence of neutralizing antibody. The neutralizing antibody titer would be taken as the serum dilution that resulted in about 25 PFU, half the number of PFUs expected simply by the dilution of the original number of PFUs, as in Table 2.2.

The neutralizing antibody in the serum completely inhibited virus replication (0 plaques were present) when minimally diluted serum (1:4 and 1:16) was used, and the 1:64 dilution largely blocked plaque

Table 2.2 Plaque-forming assay to determine neutralizing antibody titer

Tube #	Viral PFUs in 0.5 ml in each tube	Serum dilution	Volume of diluted serum added to each tube	Total volume in each tube	Number of viral PFUs in 0.1 ml of fluid of each tube, 2 plates tested per tube
#1	500	1:4	0.5 ml	1.0 ml	0/0
#2	500	1:16	0.5 ml	1.0 ml	0/0
#3	500	1:64	0.5 ml	1.0 ml	7/3
#4	500	1:256	0.5 ml	1.0 ml	22/26
#5	500	1:1,024	0.5 ml	1.0 ml	46/52

formation. At the 1:256 dilution, 22 and 26 plaques were present (an average of 24 plaques).

Investigators often use an "endpoint" of ~50% plaque reduction to indicate the antibody titer. Since 50 PFUs per 0.1 ml would be the most expected, a significant decrease from that would be sought. In this example, significant decrease would be taken as the 24 PFUs (average) with serum diluted 1:256. The neutralizing antibody titer of the serum tested would be stated to be 1:256.

However, rather than stating that the antibody titer is 1:256, the titer is often indicated to be the reciprocal, and the neutralizing antibody titer would be stated to be 256.

It is emphasized that the described measurement of neutralizing antibody titer is a bioassay. It is a time-consuming biological measurement of a type of antibody that reduces the infectivity of the particular virus used in the assay.

Not all antibody is neutralizing antibody, and antibody assays of other than neutralizing antibody can be performed. Antibody is further discussed in Chapter 4.

OTHER USES OF VIRAL PLAQUE ASSAYS

In Chapter 8 (Figure 8.1), results of a type of plaque assay used to differentiate between standard (wild-type) HSV and mutant HSV is demonstrated. The plaque assay permitted the quantitation of both virus types of viruses in a single plaque assay.

One can easily consider other uses of plaque assays. For example, varied concentrations of an antiviral might be used to determine the concentration necessary to inhibit 50% of infectious virus particles from growing in cells.

Further Reading

A Baer, K Kehn-Hall. Viral concentration determination through plaque assays using traditional and novel overlay systems. *J Vis Exp* 2014;e52065. https://doi.org/10.3791/52065

M Mendoza, K Manguiat, H Wood, M Drebot. Two detailed plaque assay protocols for the quantification of infectious SARS-CoV-2. *Curr Protoc Microbiol* 2020;**57**:ecpmc105. https://doi.org/10.1002/cpmc.105

3

Molecular Biology
The Synthesis of DNA, RNA, Protein

Aspects of molecular biology important for the replication of viral and cellular DNA and RNA genomes, and for the synthesis of proteins from RNA, are presented in this chapter. Emphasis here is on the template concept. Molecular biology discussion includes the function of genes and the mechanisms of action of antiviral medications.

The Central Dogma: The Synthesis of RNA from DNA and Protein from RNA

The Central Dogma consists of the concept of DNA being made into RNA and RNA into protein. Discoveries in the second half of the twentieth century demonstrated the means by which living things (and also viruses) reproduce. Living things consist of individual cells (bacteria, amoebas) or multiple cells (people). The initial focus here is on the processes (molecular biology and biochemistry) by which cells reproduce.

Viruses use similar processes as do living organisms in their replication. It can certainly be seen how this similarity could lead to conclusions that viruses are living organisms. However, viruses only grow in living cells and use much of the cellular biochemical processes for their replication.

The DNA of cells and the DNA of viruses are the templates for the synthesis of new cell and new viral DNA. For RNA viruses, the process is slightly modified. Most RNA viruses use their RNA as a template to make copies of their RNA, in the replication process. However, some RNA viruses use an enzyme (reverse transcriptase) to make a DNA copy of their RNA, and then make their genome RNA from that DNA copy.

RNA, specifically messenger RNA (mRNA) serves as the template for the synthesis of proteins of viruses and humans. In some RNA viruses, the RNA that serves as the template for the synthesis of new genomic RNA also serves as the mRNA template for the synthesis of proteins.[23]

Animals, including humans, are mountains of many proteins. In humans, we often talk of hemoglobin (carries oxygen to cells), insulin (necessary for sugar metabolism), muscle proteins (myoglobin), and many others. Our cells and tissues are composed of many, many different proteins. Antibodies (made by immune cells in response to infections – Chapter 4) are also proteins.

In summary, DNA is the primary means of storing genetic information, although some viruses, including SARS-CoV-2, are RNA based. The usual "Central Dogma" of DNA→RNA→protein is modified slightly for RNA viruses. All cells and viruses use mRNA as the code to make proteins. The normal Central Dogma of cell growth/replication is altered by viral infections, whereby the virus may take over the ongoing process in the infected cell.[24,25]

Three processes are considered here:

1. Replication of nucleic acid – replication of the genome
   a. Replication of DNA (deoxynucleic acid) – humans, bacteria, and DNA viruses. DNA is the template to synthesize, to replicate, the DNA genome.
   b. Replication of RNA (ribonucleic acid) – RNA viruses, for example, SARS-CoV-2. RNA is the template to synthesize the RNA genome. For some RNA viruses (human immunodeficiency virus), viral

reverse transcriptase copies the viral RNA genome into DNA, and this DNA then serves as the template to synthesize viral genome RNA.

2. Synthesis of messenger RNA (mRNA) from the DNA template – termed "transcription." Some RNA viruses use their genomic RNA as mRNA.

3. Synthesis of protein from mRNA templates – termed "translation."

While the processes of DNA replication, RNA synthesis, and protein synthesis are complex, some concepts are not. In all cases, a template is the basis – DNA to make DNA, RNA to make RNA, DNA to make mRNA, mRNA to make protein.

1.a. Replication of DNA – Human, Bacteria, DNA Viruses

DNA replication in humans is used here as an example of DNA replication.

DNA in humans exists as long strands, more specifically pairs of long strands – the double helix, two DNA strands gently wound around each other. Long stretches of DNA strands are chromosomes. Genes are parts of chromosomes.

Human cells contain 23 pairs of chromosomes. One chromosome in each pair is from the individual's mother and one from their father. These 23 pairs of chromosomes are the human genome – the DNA necessary to make a new person.

Each chromosome contains multiple genes, stretches of the DNA that are described of as "coding" for the many proteins of which we are composed.

In terms of viruses, one could think of the double-stranded DNA genome of a DNA virus such as herpes simplex virus (HSV) as the chromosome of that virus. A single strand of RNA is the genome of SARS-CoV-2.

Francis Crick, James Watson, and Maurice Wilkins received the Nobel Prize in Physiology/Medicine in 1962 for their work describing the double helix structure of human DNA. Many believe that the work of Rosalind Franklin was overlooked by the Nobel committee.

Each DNA strand is composed of chemicals termed "deoxynucleotides," which are synthesized from deoxynucleosides. Deoxynucleosides are discussed below in considering antiviral medications.

Four nucleotides, more specifically deoxynucleotides (deoxyribonucleotides), are present in DNA. Importantly, the deoxynucleotides present in one DNA strand are complementary to those in the opposite strand – they recognize and bind to the nucleotides in the opposite strand. This binding is what keeps the strands together as a double helix.

The deoxynucleotides are deoxyadenosine (dA), deoxythymidine (dT), deoxycytidine (dC), and deoxyguanosine (dG). Deoxyadenosine (dA) binds to (is complementary to) dT, and dC is complementary to dG.

Following the separation of the two strands of the double helix into two individual DNA strands, each strand serves as a template to synthesize a complementary DNA strand, resulting in two pairs of strands.

Important is the concept of complementation, which determines the sequence of the deoxynucleotides being added to the growing, new DNA strand. DNA nucleotides being added to the growing DNA strand as part of the DNA replication process are complementary to deoxynucleotides in the template strand. The end result is two original strands and a newly synthesized complementary strand for each.

The synthesis of new DNA involves the incorporation of the four deoxynucleotides into each developing DNA strand. The four nucleotides incorporated into DNA give the genetic code four possibilities at each site. The resulting possible deoxynucleotide sequences are enormous. Thus,

dA-dA-dG-dT-dC-dC-dC-dG-dG-dT-dT-dT ... dG-dG

might be a hypothetical nucleotide sequence in one DNA strand – for example, from one strand of a human double helix.

If this were the sequence of one strand of DNA, because of complementarity, the deoxynucleotide sequence of the other DNA strand in the double helix, would be

dT-dT-dC-dA-dG-dG-dG-dC-dC-dA-dA-dA ... dC-dC.

Prior to the synthesis of new DNA, the two complementary strands of DNA in the double helix are separated. Then each of the two separated strands will serve as the template for the synthesis of two new strands.

Since nucleotides such as dA and dT are complementary to one another, if dA is present in an existing DNA strand, dT will be added to a growing DNA strand opposite to dA.

Because dT binds to (is complementary to) dA and dG binds to dC. The double-stranded DNA strand would be that found in Figure 3.1.

Then, dA and dT are complementary to each other, as are dG and dC. The binding of dA to dT and of dC to dG is what connects one strand of DNA to its complementary strand in the double helix. Important is the point that either DNA strand may serve as a template to synthesize a complementary DNA strand.

Picture the two strands being bound to each other, and rather than existing simply as two lines of deoxyribonucleotides, as being gently twisted around each other – the double helix. The binding of one DNA

dA-dA-dG-dT-dC-dC-dC-dG-dG-dT-dT-dT...dG-dG   Original DNA strand

| | | | | | | | | | | | | |

dT-dT-dC-dA-dG-dG-dG-dC-dC-dA-dA-dA...dC **XX**   Newly synthesized complementary opposite DNA strand. Because of complementarity, the next deoxynucleotide to be added (**XX**) will be dC.

Figure 3.1

strand in the helix to the other is the result of them being complementary to each other.

Separation of the two strands of the double helix pair (denaturation) permits a complementary copy of each strand to be synthesized, so that two double-stranded helices result; the double stranded helix has been replicated.

The genomes of most DNA viruses are double stranded, as is human DNA, and the replication of viral DNA is similar to the replication of human DNA. The DNA synthesis of herpes simplex virus is inhibited by the antiviral medication acyclovir (a nucleoside analog). Acyclovir use results in abnormal deoxynucleotides being incorporated into HSV DNA, further discussed in Chapter 8.

The complementary nature of one strand of DNA for the other in the double helix is an important concept in discussing DNA replication in DNA-based organisms. RNA replication in most RNA viruses is similarly based on the RNA genome serving as a template for the synthesis of new RNA. RNA is composed of ribonucleotides, similar to the deoxynucleotides present in DNA.

As discussed below, specific DNA deoxynucleotides are also complementary to specific ribonucleotides of RNA. This permits the synthesis of a messenger RNA (mRNA) copy of a DNA sequence. Therefore, DNA serves as the template for the synthesis of mRNA, and mRNA serves as the template to synthesize protein. By this process, DNA genes are transcribed into mRNA, and this is translated into protein.

1.b. Replication of RNA – RNA Viruses

Replication of the RNA genome in RNA viruses is similar in concept to replication of DNA in DNA viruses, with some exceptions.

First, most RNA viruses are single stranded (SARS-CoV-2, measles virus, influenza virus). Therefore, there is no double helix to unwind, and the process is conceptually less complicated than is replication of DNA for DNA viruses.

A second difference for replication of these RNA viruses is that instead of their genome being composed of deoxynucleotides (deoxyribonucleotides), their RNA genomes are composed of ribonucleotides. Therefore, the RNA genome of an RNA virus such as SARS-CoV-2 consists of ribonucleotides, including guanosine (G)–cytidine (C)–adenine (A)–uridine (U) ... rather than deoxynucleotides such as dG-dC-dA-dT used in DNA replication.

In RNA, instead of deoxythymidine (dT) being added as the complement of dA, uridine (U) is added as the complement of dA.

An additional point in considering replication of some RNA viruses is that they first go "backwards." They make a DNA copy of their RNA genome (the DNA synthesized is complementary to the genome RNA). They then synthesize RNA from that DNA template. Therefore, the replication of their RNA genome has a complementary DNA intermediate. These viruses, such as human immunodeficiency virus (HIV) use a protein enzyme termed "reverse transcriptase" to initially make DNA from their RNA.

The "usual" sequence described in molecular biology is transcription of DNA to RNA and then translation of RNA to protein (the Central Dogma). Therefore, the initial process of RNA to DNA for HIV virus was termed to involve reverse transcription.

Nucleosides into Nucleotide

It is noted that the four deoxynucleotides in DNA are dC, dG, dA, and dT while in RNA the four ribonucleotides are C, G, A, and U. These nucleotides initially exist in cells as nucleosides. When they are phosphorylated (phosphate is added), they become nucleotides and are then incorporated into DNA or RNA. Importantly, nucleosides may readily pass into cells through the cell membrane. Nucleotides do not.

The development of antiviral medications has, in part, emphasized nucleoside analogs. These are novel nucleosides that enter cells. They are then phosphorylated, and in that form inhibit viral DNA or RNA replication. Nucleoside analogs such as acyclovir are further discussed below and in Chapter 8.

Molecular Biology Techniques

Polymerase chain reaction (PCR) technology, hybridization, and the developing methodology of antisense inhibition is discussed at this point. Important to them is the concept of complementation, which relates to the synthesis of DNA and RNA. As noted above, DNA deoxynucleotides will hybridize with (bind to) complementary DNA deoxynucleotides, and DNA deoxynucleotides will hybridize with complementary RNA ribonucleotides. Subsequent to discussion of PCR, hybridization, and antisense inhibition, we return to the Central Dogma and the synthesis of proteins from RNA.

PCR METHODOLOGY

As discussed in Chapter 1, PCR techniques have been widely discussed and extensively employed to detect SARS-CoV-2 viral RNA. The methodology utilizes the concept of complementary DNA, and so discussion of PCR fits well at this point.

Polymerase chain reaction techniques result in the great amplification of target DNA. Target DNA sequences are increased by the millions, which greatly facilitates their analysis. PCR techniques only work with DNA. Therefore, to study RNA viruses such as SARS-CoV-2, an initial step of using reverse transcriptase enzyme to make a complementary DNA copy of the target viral RNA is necessary. The synthesized complementary DNA copy is then greatly amplified.

Necessary are small DNA primer fragments (laboratory-synthesized sequences of deoxynucleotides) that are complementary to a part of the target DNA strand (therefore, the deoxynucleotide sequence of the target DNA strand need be known). In the presence of the enzyme DNA polymerase, the four canonical deoxynucleotides and the appropriate chemical conditions, the DNA strand being synthesized from the primer fragments, will be extended. A full-length complementary copy of the target DNA strand will be achieved.

With PCR amplification, from an initial single-stranded DNA target, two DNA strands will result. Next, each of these two complementary DNA strands will be used as templates to make two additional strands. The process will repeat many times, doubling the amount of target DNA with each cycle, until large amounts of the target DNA have been synthesized.

PCR cycles, typically 20–30 and each resulting in the doubling of the amount of the target DNA, are employed. The relatively large amount of DNA that is then present can then be analyzed and identified, for example, after gel electrophoresis.

Kary Mullis won the Nobel Prize in Chemistry in 1993 for his discovery of PCR methodology.

HYBRIDIZATION – BLOT HYBRIDIZATION, IN SITU HYBRIDIZATION

Hybridization was introduced in Chapter 1 in discussing the detection of viruses (Southern and northern hybridization). The straightforward concept is that probe DNA deoxynucleotides will hybridize to (bind to) target complementary deoxynucleotides. DNA deoxynucleotide probes will also hybridize to complementary ribonucleotide RNA targets.

In recent years, PCR use has increased, and blot hybridization use has decreased. One advantage of the latter over the former is that while PCR requires knowledge of the DNA deoxynucleotide sequence of the target, blot hybridization does not. However, PCR methodology is much less labor intensive than is blot hybridization, and it has become almost universal, particularly in clinical settings.

In situ hybridization is similar in concept to blot hybridization except that instead of labeled DNA binding to target complementary DNA or RNA in blots, it binds to target DNA or RNA in tissue sections. Label of the DNA probe in the tissue is evidence of the target DNA or RNA, and the cellular location of the target is also evident.

Hybridization procedures (blot and in situ) can be performed with probes of known nucleotide sequence (which is necessary for PCR) or when the DNA sequence is not known. In Chapter 5, results of in situ hybridization using a probe of known DNA sequence are presented (detection of herpes simplex virus RNA in experimental animal tissue sections). In Chapter 7, results of blot hybridization where the viral DNA sequence was not known are shown (detection of JC virus DNA from human brain).

Antisense Inhibition

The conceptual therapeutic procedure of antisense inhibition is dependent on similar probe and target nucleic acid hybridization. If probe DNA binds to target RNA in cells in tissue sections (in situ hybridization), it is only a slight stretch to consider the binding of probe DNA to target RNA in intact living individuals.

Since abnormal proteins responsible for diseases are translated from abnormal mRNAs (transcribed from abnormal DNA genes), it has been considered that a means to diminish the abnormal protein may be by inactivating the mRNA responsible for the abnormal protein. The thinking has been that DNA deoxynucleotides that readily hybridize (bind to) target mRNA in tissue sections will bind to abnormal target mRNA in individuals.

As noted, most DNA is double stranded – the double helix. A DNA gene in a cell or in a DNA virus is on what is termed the "coding strand" for that gene (also termed the "sense strand"). The DNA deoxynucleotide sequence on the opposite DNA strand is termed the "template strand" (also termed the "antisense strand"). The gene is on the coding strand (sense strand), and the template to make the mRNA is on the opposite strand (antisense strand).

To detect an mRNA, it is necessary to use the DNA sequence of the template strand, from which the mRNA was synthesized, as the probe. The DNA of the template strand is complementary to the mRNA and will hybridize to the mRNA.

Treatment with DNA fragments complementary to target mRNA to decrease protein production from that mRNA is sometimes termed "antisense inhibition." The DNA sequence of the antisense strand (the template strand) is complementary to the target mRNA and will bind to it. Since the goal is to use such antisense DNA to inhibit the mRNA, the process has been termed "antisense inhibition." This is further discussed in Chapter 9.

2. Synthesis of mRNA from the DNA Template (Transcription)

We now return to the Central Dogma, specifically the synthesis of mRNA from DNA.

The process by which mRNA (from which proteins are synthesized) is made from DNA is similar to the above concepts by which DNA is synthesized from DNA. As noted above, one strand of DNA is the template strand, which is complementary to the opposite coding DNA strand of the double helix. Complementary mRNA is synthesized from the template DNA strand by adding ribonucleotides, similar to the above process of adding deoxynucleotides for the synthesis of DNA stands.

The RNA ribonucleotides are transcribed into an mRNA strand from a DNA gene. The synthesized mRNA is a ribonucleotide copy of the deoxynucleotide DNA sequences (except that in the mRNA, uridine, U, is substituted for DNA deoxythymidine, dT). The mRNA is synthesized from the template strand that is complementary to the coding strand. Protein is then synthesized from the RNA template.

Figure 3.2 is a hypothetical example of the synthesis of mRNA as the prelude to protein synthesis.

Using the DNA sequence shown here, the complementary mRNA sequence indicated would be synthesized.

The preceding discussion directly pertains to cells and DNA viruses, which follow the Central Dogma of DNA→mRNA→protein. A slight difference in the process need be noted for RNA viruses.

The RNA of some RNA viruses (for example, SARS-CoV-2) serves as the mRNA from which proteins are made. These are termed "positive-sense RNA viruses." Other positive-sense RNA viruses include poliovirus and West Nile virus. The viral RNA serves as the mRNA template from which proteins are made, and the RNA is also copied for viral RNA genome replication.[25]

In negative-sense RNA viruses, the RNA also serves as the genome of the virus. However, rather than the genome RNA also serving as mRNA (as it does for positive-sense RNA viruses), mRNA is synthesized from the viral genome RNA. That synthesized mRNA then serves as the template

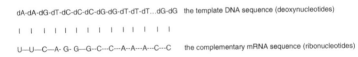

dA-dA-dG-dT-dC-dC-dC-dG-dG-dT-dT-dT...dG-dG   the template DNA sequence (deoxynucleotides)

| | | | | | | | | | | | |

U—U—C—A· G· G—G--C---C---A--A---A---C---C   the complementary mRNA sequence (ribonucleotides)

Figure 3.2

for protein synthesis. Examples of negative-sense RNA viruses are measles virus, rabies virus, and influenza virus.

3. Synthesis of Protein from mRNA Templates (Translation), the Final Step of the Central Dogma Process

The synthesis of a protein (a string of many amino acids) from an mRNA template strand is similar in concept to synthesizing DNA or RNA from a template. One difference, however, is that groups of three mRNA ribonucleotides, for example, C-A-C, are "read" to indicate an amino acid. Instead of a single nucleotide "selecting" its complementary ribonucleotide or deoxynucleotide, a group of three ribonucleotides "selects" an amino acid.

Each such group of three mRNA ribonucleotides, termed a "codon," codes for an amino acid. For example, the mRNA nucleotide triplet of C-A-C codes for the amino acid histidine. Therefore, C-A-C on an mRNA strand will result in the amino acid histidine being added to an elongating chain of amino acids on its way to becoming a protein.

At present, 20 amino acids (of the more than 250 that are known to exist in nature) have been described as being coded for by mRNAs and are added to one another in growing amino acid chains, which leads to protein formation.

CENTRAL DOGMA SUMMARY – DNA→RNA→PROTEIN

Deoxynucleotide sequences of DNA strands are transcribed into complementary mRNA. The mRNA is then translated into individual amino acids, which when linked in appropriate sequence form proteins.

The preceding discussions of the synthesis and replication of DNA and RNA and the synthesis of protein form a descriptive overview of very complex processes. Much complexity is necessary, including accurate signals of where to start and stop the process for each gene. However, not difficult to follow are the concepts of using a template strand of deoxynucleotides (DNA) to synthesize a copy of itself – replication of the DNA genome; using a template strand of DNA to synthesize an RNA copy of the DNA; and using the RNA copy as a template to synthesize a protein.

Genes

In the long strands of genomic DNA or RNA, specific stretches (sequences) of DNA deoxynucleotides (DNA viruses, humans) or stretches of RNA (RNA viruses) are genes. As noted above, the DNA sequences lead to the transcription of complementary-specific mRNA ribonucleotide sequences, and the translation of these mRNA sequences leads to the construction of specific amino acid sequences, that is, proteins.

Also as noted, the process is slightly different for RNA viruses but conceptually similar – ribonucleotide sequences (genes) serve as the templates for the synthesis of proteins.

Discussion of humans is generally of our DNA genes responsible for all of our proteins.

Human genes are responsible for blood types A, B, and O. People have the A protein (they are blood type A), the B protein (type B), both A and B proteins (type AB), or neither protein (type O). These were the first human protein polymorphisms described, and Karl Landsteiner won the Nobel Prize in Physiology/Medicine in 1930 for the discovery.

It is common for a given protein to vary slightly among people (protein polymorphism), similar to the polymorphisms of the ABO system. In discussions of the immune system in Chapter 4, a number of proteins important for combating infections are noted. It is very likely that polymorphisms exist among the proteins in this system, and it is likely that some protein variants may prove to be important for resistance to particular viral infections.

It is of interest that some reports have suggested that people with blood type O might be slightly less likely to be infected with SARS-CoV-2. If proved to be true, this may be a fruitful area of investigation.

Although variation of specific amino acids in particular proteins (polymorphisms) are common and often not harmful, sometimes they are harmful. Sometimes, if a single deoxynucleotide in the DNA of a gene is incorrect, the result may result in an incorrect mRNA, therefore an incorrect amino acid, and therefore an abnormal and harmful protein.

For example, sickle cell disease results from the normal dG-dA-dG sequence in the beta-globin gene DNA being changed to abnormal dG-dT-dG. When transcribed to mRNA and then translated to the hemoglobin protein, this results in the amino acid valine being substituted for the amino acid glutamic acid. This single deoxynucleotide change results in an amino acid change, and this results in a severe illness.

Real progress is being made in correcting this mutation by using a virus to deliver the normal beta-globin gene to the cells of sickle cell disease patients.[26]

Such therapy is an example of using a virus to deliver therapeutic DNA to cells, relying on the ability of viruses to enter cells. These viruses are modified to incorporate the DNA gene of interest, and also so that they do not cause disease. Virus vectors that have been used in such treatments have included retrovirus, adenovirus, adeno-associated virus, and herpes simplex virus. This is further discussed in Chapter 9.

Dominant vs Recessive Mutations

Human clinical mutations such as those that cause sickle cell disease occur because of abnormalities in genes. Genetic abnormalities result, often discussed as being autosomal dominant, autosomal recessive, and X-linked recessive genetic abnormalities.

AUTOSOMAL DOMINANT

Clinical illness occurs if the mutation is present on one autosomal chromosome (of the chromosome pair), even though the other autosomal chromosome (of the pair) is normal. Examples are Huntington's disease and polycystic kidney disease. These may be transmitted by an abnormal gene of one parent, even if the other parent does not have the abnormality.

AUTOSOMAL RECESSIVE

Clinical illness occurs if the mutation is present on both chromosomes (of the chromosome pair). Examples are sickle cell disease and cystic fibrosis. These are transmitted by receiving the abnormal gene from both parents.

X-LINKED RECESSIVE

Clinical illness occurs in males who have the mutation on the X chromosome they received from their mothers. Their mothers who have a second normal X chromosome do not have the clinical illness, although they are carriers of the illness. Daughters will have received a normal X chromosome from their fathers. They will have a 50:50 chance of receiving the abnormal X chromosome from their mothers, and so they will have a 50:50 chance of being carriers.

The Importance of 3-Dimensional Structure

Before leaving molecular biology, it is important to consider the role of the 3-dimensional structure of amino acids and proteins. The 3-dimensionality of amino acids and proteins has great importance in considering how proteins function, including how antibodies that protect against viruses (and other pathogens) are made and perform their antiviral functions. Proteins consist of sequences of amino acids, but they are not simply strings of letters.

For example, a molecule of the amino acid valine may be chemically written in 1 dimension as $C_5H_{11}NO_2$, in terms of the numbers of its carbon, hydrogen, nitrogen, and oxygen atoms. Or it could be written as a 2-dimensional structure, as shown in Figure 3.3.

The 3-dimensional structure of proteins may be as important as the amino acid sequence in determining protein function.

The 3-dimensional structure is not easily indicated, but is very important, for example, for the binding of a protein to a receptor. Consider a key being placed into the keyhole of a lock. The 3-dimensional structures of both are important.

Similarly, the 3-dimensional structures of antibodies and antigens is important. Antibodies are proteins made by cells, and these recognize the

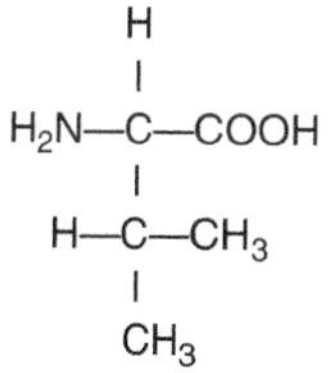

This 2-dimensional representation does more justice to the molecule as it exists in nature. But to really do it justice, picture the H_2N group (bold) projecting out of the plane of the page. Then picture a protein consisting of a string of 100 or more amino acids, each with chemical groups, some projecting out of the plane of the page and some behind the plane of the page.

Figure 3.3

3-dimensional structure of virus proteins (antigens), for example, when antibody is made against SARS-CoV-2 virus. This will be important in the next chapter, which outlines immunology, particularly the synthesis of antibodies.

The 3-dimensional structure will be important when discussing prions in Chapter 7.

Epigenetics

The preceding discussion of the Central Dogma outlines the process by which genes (sequences of DNA or RNA) are translated into proteins. Proteins are the primary building blocks of individuals and are the primary components of the physiological functions of individuals. Proteins are everything. And in all of us they start with our DNA genes. The DNA genes an individual is born with are the genes they express throughout their life. Except, this is not always true. Sometimes, some genes while present are "turned off." If a gene coding for a specific protein is turned off, that protein will not be produced.

It is easy to consider the genes of identical twins as being the same, but also to consider that a gene of one twin may be "turned off," to explain differences in illness between them. Understanding such occurrences may be important in the understanding of mechanisms by which individuals combat infections, including viral infections.

Epigenetics is the new and rapidly developing science of understanding the mechanisms by which genes are turned on or off.[27] Epigenetics is further discussed in Chapter 9.

Antiviral Medications

Recent developments of antiviral medications have often been predicated on the molecular biology of viruses.

Antiviral medications have been difficult to develop, in part because viruses grow/replicate only within cells, and they use cellular functions. Medications that inhibit viruses might very likely also inhibit cellular functioning. However, great progress has been made, with emphasis in recent years on the development of antivirals to treat HIV infections. Medications that have been developed include those that impair viral RNA synthesis (nucleoside analogs) and those that impair viral protein synthesis (protease inhibitors).

HERPES SIMPLEX VIRUS (HSV)

Possibly the first true antiviral was acyclovir, used to treat HSV infections. Acyclovir was developed in 1974 and is a nucleoside analog of thymidine (dT). It is effective in the treatment of herpes simplex virus and varicella-zoster virus. After modification in the virus-infected cell, acyclovir inhibits the viral DNA polymerase, resulting in impaired viral DNA genome synthesis. Acyclovir was the first specific antiviral, and Gertrude Elion won the Nobel Prize in Physiology/Medicine in 1988, in part for its development. Details of the mechanisms by which acyclovir inhibits HSV replication are discussed in Chapter 8.

The success of acyclovir led to the development of other nucleoside analogs.[28,29]

SARS-CoV-2

Nucleoside analog antivirals under development to treat SARS-CoV-2 infection include remdesivir, molnupiravir, and nirmatrelvir. Their usefulness in the treatment of COVID-19 patients remains to be more fully elucidated.

Remdesivir is an analog of the nucleoside adenosine, and when phosphorylated to the nucleotide form has antiviral activity. It is incorporated into the growing viral RNA genome strand of RNA viruses, and the abnormal nucleotide blocks continuing replication of the RNA strand.

Remdesivir use has been investigated in the treatment of several RNA virus infections, including SARS-CoV-2. It seems effective in the treatment of infection by Middle East respiratory coronavirus (MERS-CoV). It is promising but too early to know where it will fit in the control of SARS-CoV-2.

Molnupiravir is an analog of the nucleoside cytidine. After phosphorylation to the nucleotide form, it impairs function of the viral RNA polymerase. It had been investigated as a potential anti-influenza drug. Recently, there has been much interest in it as an anti-SARS-CoV-2 medication, where effectiveness has been demonstrated.

Nirmatrelvir is another type of antiviral medication being investigated for the treatment of SARS-CoV-2. It is a viral protease inhibitor, which class of medications has had great promise in the treatment of human immunodeficiency virus (HIV).

Nucleoside analogs and protease inhibitors have both been successfully used in the treatment of HIV infections. With both HIV and SARS-CoV-2 being RNA viruses, it is likely much information obtained in recent years to treat the former will be applicable in treating the latter.

HEPATITIS

Lamivudine, an analog of cytidine, has been used to treat hepatitis B and HIV infection.

HUMAN IMMUNODEFICIENCY VIRUS (HIV)

As noted above, several antivirals have been developed to treat HIV infections.

Azidothymidine (AZT) is a thymidine nucleoside analog and was the first effective medications for the treatment of HIV infection. It inhibits the HIV reverse transcriptase and thereby inhibits viral replication.

Other nucleoside analogs have been developed to treat HIV infections, such as didanosine, an analog of adenosine, and abacavir, an analog of guanidine. Many additional nucleoside analogs and non-nucleoside analogs have been developed to treat HIV infection (Chapter 5). Combinations of medications have been developed, in part to decrease the issue of drug resistance that may occur when a single medication is administered.

The development of antiviral medications received a big boost with the focus and efforts that resulted from the acquired immunodeficiency disease syndrome (AIDS) pandemic, caused by HIV. It is likely there will be a similar increase in antiviral medication development as a result of the COVID-19 pandemic.

The above overview touches on antiviral treatment, and discussion of antivirals will return to consider a viral mutant resistant to antiviral medication in Chapter 8.

MITOCHONDRIAL MYOPATHY

An occasional side effect noted in some HIV patients treated with AZT was damage to mitochondria and the development of "mitochondrial myopathy." Other medications have also been noted to damage mitochondria.[30]

Mitochondria are intracellular organelles that are primarily thought of as the energy-producing part of cells. They generate adenosine triphosphate (ATP), the primary energy source of cells.

Mitochondria are thought of as "endosymbionts" by some investigators. Very briefly, they are thought to once have been free-living organisms that millennia ago became incorporated into cells,[31] to the mutual advantage of the mitochondria and of the cells. Interestingly, mitochondria contain DNA by which they replicate in cells. They have their own "genome." This would seem to support the concept that they were once free-living organisms. Endosymbionts are further considered in Chapter 6, in discussions of endogenous retroviruses.

Mitochondria are interesting for another reason – they are all obtained from the individual's mother. That is, all of the mitochondria in all of my cells were obtained from my mother. Mitochondria were in the ovum from which I was conceived, and those mitochondria generated all of the mitochondria in all of my cells. Implicit in the statement that "those mitochondria generated all of the mitochondria in my cells" is the second very interesting feature of mitochondria. As noted above, these intracellular organelles contain DNA, and they replicate themselves.

On occasion AZT used to treat HIV infection was found to impair mitochondrial replication in cells, resulting in clinical illness. This disorder sometimes went by the name "mitochondrial myopathy," since muscle impairment was frequent, but other tissues, particularly other parts of the nervous system, were also involved.

AZT is a nucleoside analog antiviral, and after being phosphorylated in cells to the active antiviral form, it inhibits the replication of HIV. It does this by interfering with the viral reverse transcriptase, the enzyme that copies the viral RNA into a complementary DNA copy. As described above, this process of "reverse transcription" is necessary for the replication of HIV. However, phosphorylated AZT may interfere with mitochondrial DNA replication, resulting in mitochondrial myopathy.

Phosphorylation of AZT to the active form in cells is performed by the cellular enzyme thymidine kinase (TK). Termed "cytosolic TK" or "TK1," this TK is different from the TK2 of mitochondria, which is important for the replication of mitochondria. Discussion of TK is introduced at this time in part as prelude to further consideration of cellular TK and discussion of an important TK coded for by a virus (Chapter 8).

Further Reading

P Arbuthnot, MS Weinberg. *Applied RNA: From Fundamental Research to Therapeutic Applications*, Caister Academic Press, 2014. Book 9781908230430, E-book 9781908230676

R Chaudhry, K Khaddour. *Biochemistry, DNA Replication*, Stat Pearls, 2022. www.ncbi .nlm.nih.gov/books/NBK482125/

4

The Immune System
Innate and Adaptive

Following viral infection, viral replication proceeds. The infected individual will mount an immune response to control the infection.

The immune system is often divided into the innate immune system and the adaptive immune system. The innate system includes proteins termed "cytokines," which are released by cells drawn to sites of infection or injury. These proteins are released early after infection and are not specific for the type of infection. They may upregulate, or sometimes downregulate, aspects of the adaptive immune system.

The Adaptive System develops after immune cells are "educated." It takes a longer period of time before it is manifest than does the innate system, and it is specific for the type of infection. A significant part of the adaptive system is the synthesis of antibodies. Antibodies are proteins made against protein antigens including of viruses such as SARS-CoV-2. They are specific for individual viruses and, more particularly, for parts of viruses (for example, the spikes of SARS-CoV-2). Even more specifically, when made against viral proteins such as SARS-CoV-2 spikes, they are made against parts of the spikes. The part of the antigen (the part of the spike protein) to which antibody is made is termed the epitope.

The inflammatory response to viral infections is complex.[32,33] Not only is the response important for protection against infection by various types of pathogens, it is important in protection against cancer. Sometimes abnormalities in the immune system lead to autoimmune illnesses, when the immune system attacks/damages normal cells. In the brief summary to follow, only some of the components of the innate immune system are listed, and emphasis is on aspects of the adaptive immune system, particularly the development of antibody.

Innate Immune System

The innate immune system consists of a large number of proteins that may be released in response to infection or injury.

Cytokines – synthesized by multiple cell types (some cytokines may be involved in autoimmune illnesses)

Interferons – multiple types

Interleukins – many types

Tumor necrosis factors – multiple types

Complement System – many components

Many of the innate immune system proteins, including interferons and other cytokines vary slightly among groups of people. These variations, protein polymorphisms, may have important roles in one illness or another, and they are likely important in considering the varied response to illnesses among people.

Many protein polymorphisms are known in humans. As noted in Chapter 3, the first protein polymorphism system noted in humans was the ABO blood system. The possible clinical effects of the polymorphisms of many human proteins, including those of the innate immune system largely remain to be determined.

Some patients with COVID-19 infections worsen due to what is sometimes termed the "cytokine storm," the excessive or inappropriate release of components of the innate immune system, resulting in excessive inflammation. Anti-inflammatory medications such as corticosteroids are often used to treat this.[34] In considering the treatment of a viral illness such as COVID-19, it is necessary to differentiate between treatments to decrease viral replication, for example, with antivirals

(Chapters 3, 8), and treatment with disease-modifying medications, such as corticosteroids, to decrease inflammation.

There has been much discussion on the treatment of SARS-CoV-2 cytokine storm, which sometimes is more significant than is the viral infection itself. The corticosteroid dexamethasone is useful to treat inflammation, and aspirin for the Kawasaki-like illness in children may be useful. Hydroxychloroquine is not a good choice.

The release and effects of specific cytokines among people may explain why some people do well after different viral illnesses and why others have a more severe course. Polymorphisms among proteins important for immunity may be important for disease control.[33]

Worsening of patients with multiple sclerosis has been noted after treatment with cytokines such as interferon gamma and treatment with tumor necrosis factor inhibitors (Chapter 7).

Interferons

Interestingly, interferons were so named because in laboratory studies they were noted to "interfere" with viral replication. Three types of human interferons have been described: Type I (including alpha and beta), Type II (gamma), and Type III. Alpha interferon has been used to treat patients with hepatitis B and hepatitis C. Beta interferon has been used to treat patients with multiple sclerosis. The interferons have multiple actions, and it is difficult to predict efficacy in viral infections such as the COVID-19 pandemic.

For example, consider beta interferon treatment of individuals with multiple sclerosis, effective as an immunomodulatory agent although it remains unclear as to its specific mechanism. It has been possible for investigators to evaluate SARS-CoV-2 infections in multiple sclerosis patients who were being treated with beta interferon. No significant antiviral clinical effect has been noted.

Complement System

There are 50 or more proteins which "complement" the immune system, the complement system. The proteins of this system are typically activated by complexes of antibody (for example, antibody to a virus) and antigen (the virus). Subsequent to antibody binding to antigen, complement may expedite clearing of the virus. Complement components also increase inflammation by the attraction of inflammatory cells.

Antibody, part of the adaptive immune system (discussed below) is commonly measured, but the many components of the innate immune system are not. Not only is the possible clinical importance of polymorphisms among complement and the other cytokines difficult to determine, it is difficult to determine the possible importance of the amounts of these components of the innate immune system in disease pathogenesis.

Adaptive Immune System

Human blood contains red cells and white cells. The latter are important in the adaptive immune system, and lymphocytes are the type of white blood cells probably most important in the control of viral infections.

WHITE BLOOD CELLS IN HUMANS

Neutrophils ~60% of peripheral blood white cells – They are particularly important in control of infection by bacteria and fungi.

Eosinophils ~2% – They are important in control of infection by parasites.

Basophils ~0.5% – They are important for histamine release.

Monocytes ~5% – They are important in removing dead cells, and in the initial release of cytokines.

Lymphocytes ~30% – They are important in control of viral infections and cancer control.

T LYMPHOCYTES (T CELLS)

CD 4 – helper T cells. When stimulated they release cytokines (Innate Immune System) which enhance CD 8 T cell activity. They also enhance antibody production by B lymphocytes.

CD 8 – cytotoxic T cells. These cells kill virus-infected and cancer cells and release cytokines. They are most effective when stimulated by CD 4 T cells.

T_{Reg} – regulatory T cells. These cells are important for "tolerance," whereby the normal tissue cells of an individual are not rejected. They are important for such self-tolerance and what has been termed immune homeostasis. T_{Reg} cells are important in preventing autoimmune illnesses and may release inhibitory cytokines which limit inflammation.

These cells are also important in cancer control. Several medications (monoclonal antibodies) such as pembrolizumab, atezolizumab, nivolumab, and ipilimumab are effective through enhancing T cell control of tumors. It is thought that T_{Reg} lymphocytes lose the ability to immunologically limit cancer growth because of cancer cell expression of immune checkpoint proteins. The therapeutic monoclonals block those proteins, resulting in increased immune antitumor reactivity.

In brief, T_{Reg} cells, may be underactive in autoimmune illnesses and overactive in cancer, resulting in excessive immune inflammation in the former and decreased immunological control in the latter.

NK (natural killer cells) – These lymphocytes have actions that are analogous to those of CD 8 lymphocytes. They typically respond more quickly than do CD 8 cells, usually in response to cytokines such as interferons.

B lymphocytes (B cells) – These lymphocytes make antibody (immunoglobulin [Ig], termed gamma globulin in older literature). Publications have sometimes referred to mature antibody-producing B cells as plasma cells or plasma B cells. B cells make several types of Ig.

Types of Ig

Immunoglobulin A (IgA) – The prominent Ig released by B cells that are present in mucous membranes (mouth, eyes, gastrointestinal tract).

IgD – A minor Ig.

IgE – Important in immunity to parasites (for example). Increased amounts are found in people with allergies.

IgG – Discussed below.

IgM – Discussed below.

T Cells: Cell-Mediated Immunity

As noted above, the adaptive immune system includes several types of T cells (T lymphocytes), and these cells are important in virus control. However, their antiviral functions are much more difficult to measure than is B cell activity, typically performed by the measurement of antibody.

It is likely that laboratory measures of T cell antiviral function will be enhanced in the future,[35] and this will provide a more complete understanding of antiviral defenses. This will be an important area of development.

T cells are activated by foreign protein antigens. However, these antigens need to be presented by cells (for example, B cells) to the T cells in conjunction with other proteins on the surface of the antigen presenting cells. These other proteins are components of the major histocompatibility complex (MHC) which are present on cells. MHC proteins are often referred to as transplantation antigens and are discussed in organ transplant situations, where the MHC "match" between the donor and the recipient is emphasized.

Antigen presenting cells need present the foreign protein (for example, viral protein such as SARS-CoV-2 spike protein) to T lymphocytes in conjunction with the appropriate MHC proteins. This complex procedure makes the measurement of T cell reactivity to, for example, SARS-CoV-2 spike proteins more difficult than measuring antibody (Ig) to the spikes, the product of B cells.

Peter Doherty and Rolf Zinkernagel won the Nobel Prize in Physiology/Medicine in 1996 for their work on how T lymphocytes recognize antigens in conjunction with MHC recognition.

An example of a human test of T cell reactivity, sometimes termed "delayed hypersensitivity" (type IV hypersensitivity), is tuberculosis (tb) skin testing. This was widely performed in the past for the diagnosis of tb. To perform the test, a small amount of tb material was injected into the skin. A positive test consisted of the development of an area of swelling, redness (erythema) several days later (that is, delayed in time from the time of the injection). The area of inflammation is thought to be the result primarily of CD 8 T lymphocytes that recognized the injected tb protein.

As compared with measuring B cell activity by measuring antibody in a test tube, such measuring of T cell activity is considerably more difficult. To test for antibody, the individual (human or animal) from whom the antibody came is not important.

Significant progress in T cell measurement is occurring, in part related to the COVID-19 pandemic. For example, it is becoming possible to identify T cells that recognize specific SARS-CoV-2 protein antigens. In these studies, white blood cells are isolated from patients and exposed to SARS-CoV-2 virus. Some of the T cells that recognize the virus produce interferon gamma as a result of their being activated by the virus, and these cells can be quantitated.

In addition, investigations of the role(s) of T_{Reg} lymphocytes in autoimmune illnesses and in cancer control have been greatly expanded recently. It would be of interest to determine a possible role of T_{Reg} lymphocytes in the inflammatory response to viral infections.

Emphasis in further discussion of the adaptive immune system will be on the B cell antibody response, because of the great interest in antibody as a means to diagnose prior infection by SARS-CoV-2, as a means to measure the efficacy of vaccines, and the possible use of antibody to treat infection by that virus. However, T lymphocyte reactivity may prove to be of great importance in SARS-CoV-2 control, including after immunization.

B Cells: Humoral Immunity

Antibodies are immunoglobulin (Ig) proteins. There are several classes of Igs (IgA-IgM), and at any point in time, humans have many different antibodies throughout their bodies.

After a viral infection, the emphasis in Ig antibody production by B cells is on IgM and IgG, and to a lesser degree IgA. The present discussion focuses on IgM and IgG, usually discussed in terms of testing for evidence of a viral infection, and in considering protection from against a virus after immunization.

When a B cell "recognizes" an antigen epitope (a part of a specific viral protein, including its 3-dimensional structure), it starts to make Ig antibody. Initially, the B cell synthesizes IgM, which will bind to that antigen epitope. After a period of time, the B cell switches to making IgG to that epitope.

Gerald Edelman and Rodney Porter won the Nobel Prize in Physiology/Medicine in 1972 for their work on the structure of Ig molecules.

In practice, if Ig antibody to a viral protein antigen that is detected in the blood of a patient is only of the IgM class, it is concluded that the infection was recent. With time, IgM to that viral antigen will no longer be produced, and IgG to the same viral antigen will be produced by that B cell. There will be an overlap period when IgM and IgG to the viral antigen are both detectable. Later, only IgG to the antigen will be detectable, often lifelong.

If in the future the individual is reinfected with the same virus, IgM antibody may again be produced. IgM antibody may also be produced if a latent virus infection in an individual is reactivated. Such reactivation and IgM antibody production is discussed for BK virus reactivation during pregnancy (Chapter 7).

IgG will cross the placenta. Therefore, when a woman delivers a baby, that infant will have the IgG antibodies of the mother and will be protected against specific infections. However, the infant will not have the B cells that synthesized the IgG in the mother (which the mother continues to have), and so those IgG levels (and infection protection) will decrease with time. IgG in the infant that was acquired from the mother will decrease by ~50% per month.

This half-life of IgG also is the same when treating patients with antibody, either monoclonal or polyclonal (discussed below). Of course, as part of their care, infants are routinely immunized against several pathogens, and this stimulates their own B cells, and long-term protection results.

The recognition by a B lymphocyte of a specific antigenic site of a protein (the epitope) is the start of the process. As noted previously, the amino acid sequence of the protein is important for the recognition process, and the 3-dimensional structure of the protein is important in the epitope configuration. It is not the entire protein that is recognized by the B cell, but only a part, the epitope.

Different epitopes of multiple viral protein antigens are recognized by different B cells. Polyclonal antibody is the result of the Ig produced by the many different B cells. Each lymphocyte makes Ig to only one epitope of one protein antigen. That is the crux of monoclonal antibody.

POLYCLONAL ANTIBODY

Since many different B cells will recognize different epitopes of many different proteins, for example, spikes of SARS-CoV-2, many different antibodies to the virus will be produced – polyclonal antibody.

Consider B cells that recognize and make antibody to the spikes on SARS-CoV-2. The spikes are proteins and consist of amino acids, with a 3-dimensional form. Hypothetically, consider that part of a spike protein consists of the amino acid sequence valine-valine-isoleucine-leucine, abbreviated as V-V-I-L. Picture that a specific B cell might recognize the top of the sequence, for example, the top half of each letter. That is the epitope to which it responds. Another B cell might recognize the bottom of the letters. Therefore, the B cells will have recognized and will make antibody to different epitopes, different parts, of the same protein antigen.

Many B cells will make Ig antibody to various spike protein epitopes. Other B cells will make antibody to other viral protein antigens (other epitopes). All of the Ig antibody made in response to recognition of the many viral antigen epitopes by the many B cells is polyclonal antibody. When individuals are infected with a virus or other pathogen and then recover, they will have in their blood all of these antibodies. If their blood containing these antibodies is given to another individual to treat infection by the virus, the recipient will have received polyclonal antibody.

MONOCLONAL ANTIBODY

The many antibodies produced by many B cells to many epitopes will be of different quality, for example, in their ability to neutralize (inactivate) the virus to which they were produced. It is possible with modern technology to isolate particular individual B cells that make high-quality antibody. Those individual B cells can be grown in almost limitless amounts, and the high-quality antibody they produce can be made in almost limitless amounts. Ig antibody from a particular B cell (a B cell clone) is monoclonal antibody. And it can be administered to patients.

Monoclonal antibodies, including combinations of monoclonal antibodies, are being tested in COVID-19 patients. For example, REGN-CoV-2 is a mixture of two monoclonal antibodies, each of which has good neutralizing antibody potential, casirivimab and imdevimab. And AZD7442 is a combination of tixagevimab and cilgavimab. A monoclonal antibody approved to treat COVID-19 patients is bebtelovimab.

Polyclonal[36] and monoclonal[37] antibody therapies have been considered in the treatment of COVID-19 patients. However, as forms of passive immunization, they would be of diminished value after 1 month, although their administration might be repeated.

Many monoclonal antibodies are being developed to treat many types of illnesses. Several used to alter T_{Reg} lymphocyte function in the treatment of cancer patients were noted above.

Antibody Testing

Multiple methods can be used to test for Ig antibody, for example, in an individual after clinical SARS-CoV-2 infection, or after having received a vaccine. The available vaccines are very effective in raising antibody levels to the virus. However, it is difficult to determine, based on the antibody titer alone, the degree to which the person would be protected against subsequent infection. Currently available methods do not test for memory B lymphocytes or T lymphocytes. And while most would agree that a higher antibody titer is likely to be more protective than a lower titer, specifics are slight.[5]

For the most part, antibody, measured against a virus after viral illness or after the administration of a vaccine is IgG antibody, and less frequently IgM. As noted above, IgM antibody to the antigen is initially produced, followed after a period of time by IgG to the antigen. Both IgG and IgM can be measured with varied methods.

Since multiple methods to measure serum IgG and IgM antibody exist, important in comparing antibody levels over time in an individual is that the same method be used each time. Varied methods use different endpoints and report results using different units. For example, an antibody titer determined by ELISA testing (discussed below) would likely be different from a neutralizing antibody titer (Chapter 2). Since antibody measuring methods are generally biological assays, varied methods will likely result in different titers.

The titer of an antibody to, for example, SARS-CoV-2 is not the amount of IgG present as chemically measured, but rather the highest dilution (the most dilute serum), which results in a previously determined endpoint. Antibody titer determinations are bioassays and not chemical assays. Increased amounts of chemically determined IgG in multiple sclerosis is discussed in Chapter 7.

The titer of an antibody is usually indicated as the highest dilution of serum that gives a predetermined positive result. For example, if serum which is diluted to 1:1,024 (one part serum and 1,023 parts diluent) is the most dilute serum of an individual that neutralizes 50% of the infectious virus present, the neutralizing antibody titer would be 1:1,024. As discussed in Chapter 2, instead of the titer being stated to be 1:1,024, it is common practice to describe the titer as the reciprocal of 1:1,024, that is 1,024.

Most testing of antibody has been performed by the serial dilution of the serum being tested. The highest (greatest) dilution that still provides a positive result is the titer of that antibody in the serum. Multiple methods are being investigated to try to minimize the need for testing serial dilutions. Ideal would be the measurement of antibody to a virus in undiluted serum using methods that are as objective as the measuring of substances in blood, such as the serum sodium.

At present, many types of biological assays exist that measure antibody. Several are discussed in what follows.

IMMUNOHISTOCHEMISTRY

Methods of antibody testing include determination of antibody binding to cells, for example, binding of IgG against SARS-CoV-2 to cells infected with the virus. Throat swab cells that bind antibody to the virus would be evidence of COVID-19. Rather than relying on polymerase chain reaction (PCR) detection of SARS-CoV-2 RNA as indicating infection, the presence of viral antigen would be evidence of infection. Immunohistochemistry methodology is often used to identify whether an antigen such as viral protein is present in a tissue specimen (for example, Figure 1.1, Chapter 1).

Immunohistochemistry methods are usually used to detect viral antigen in tissue and not to measure antibody levels in serum. However, by testing dilutions of serum and using known virus infected tissue, it is possible to measure the titer, the amount of antibody in serum. For example, if a label, such as in Figure 1.1, were present with human serum diluted 1:256 but not with the same serum diluted 1:1,024, it would be concluded that the titer, as determined by that method, is 1:256 (that is, 256). It is again emphasized that different methods of antibody measurement often result in different titers.

As discussed in Chapter 1, labeled antibody may be used to detect viral antigen. More commonly unlabeled antibody (primary antibody) is used – which binds to the viral antigen –followed by labeled antibody (secondary antibody), which binds to the primary antibody.

LATERAL FLOW TECHNOLOGY

As discussed in Chapter 1, lateral flow technology is a methodology to detect the presence of a viral (or another antigen). Commercial antibody is supplied, and so while it may be useful to detect viral antigen in an individual, for example, viral antigen in a nasopharyngeal swab, it is not used to determine antibody in individuals. It is similar to immunohistochemistry in that known antibody is used to detect possible viral antigen.

ELISA

Enzyme-linked immunoassay (ELISA) testing is the most automated means to measure antibody in individuals and is commonly performed. Typically, in multiple wells of a plastic tray, SARS-CoV-2 antigen is added, which binds to the plastic of the wells. A series of serum dilutions from a patient is then added. If antibody to the virus is present in the serum of the patient, it will bind to the viral antigens. This binding antibody is termed the "primary antibody."

A secondary antibody against human IgG is then added. The secondary antibody would have, for example, peroxidase bound to it. A colorant would be added to detect the presence of the peroxidase. Color in the fluid would be read. The most dilute serum that still gives a color signal would be taken as the antibody titer.

The procedure described is the common indirect method (using a primary antibody and a secondary antibody to the first antibody, which is labeled). Alternatively, a direct method, using a primary antibody that is labeled may be used. Other variations on ELISA testing exist, including the capture method discussed in Chapter 1.

NEUTRALIZING ANTIBODY

Neutralizing antibody titer can be determined by plaque assay. As discussed in Chapter 2, given amounts of virus (known numbers of plaque-forming units [PFUs]) are put in multiple tubes. To each tube, increasing dilutions of serum from a patient are added. The neutralizing antibody titer will be determined by the degree to which PFUs are decreased by the antibody. The greatest dilution (the most dilute serum) that still gives the endpoint of inhibiting ~50% of the PFUs would be taken as the neutralizing antibody titer. The concept of neutralizing antibody titer has an attraction in that it suggests protection.

Antibody measurement by any of several methods is not difficult, although the interpretation may not be so straightforward. That is, the amount and type of antibody important to minimize subsequent infection are not clear.[5]

DURATION OF ANTIBODY RESPONSE

Individuals will have antibodies of varying titers to antigens when they are immunized with a viral vaccine or after recovery from viral infections. In either case, they mount an active immune response. While the duration of the antibody response varies among illnesses and vaccines, the duration will be greater than after passive immunization. As noted above, there are multiple methods to measure antibody, and in comparing antibody levels over time in an individual, it is important to use the same method for each measurement.

After passive immunization, such as receiving polyclonal or monoclonal antibody, the amount of antibody will decrease by ~50% per month. As noted above, since IgG crosses the placenta, newborn infants will have antibody from their mothers. In effect, they have been passively immunized.

Recipients of passive immunization do not receive memory B lymphocytes or T lymphocytes as part of the immunization process, while individuals who, for example, overcome clinical SARS-CoV-2 illness or who receive a SARS-CoV-2 vaccine would likely have these cells. They may have decreased antibody with time, but more difficult to measure immune cellular functions may be paramount in minimizing future illness.

An interesting hypothetical experiment to perform would be to compare viral infection protection in two groups of individuals with equivalent antibody titers, one group with antibody as a result of passive immunization and the other with antibody as a result of active immunization. Individuals in the former group would have antibody without any potentially antiviral T lymphocytes, and those in the latter group would have antibody as well as potential antiviral T lymphocytes.

Viral Vaccines

It is possible to imagine how in the past, people recognized that individuals who recovered from an infection seemed to be protected from getting that illness again. From this, it is likely that the earliest use of material from sick patients was to try to prevent disease in others. The first well-defined vaccine preparation was by Edward Jenner in 1796. He treated people with cowpox material (from cow infections) to protect against the related smallpox virus.

However, before that time people had practiced variolation – using tissue from people who had smallpox (variola) to prevent against smallpox in others. It likely was first used in China. Smallpox scab material was used to for skin inoculation and made into snuff-like material that was given intranasally.

As an interesting aside, smallpox was differentiated from the great pox (syphilis). The last case of smallpox is said to have occurred in 1977. It was concluded in 1980 by the World Health Organization that smallpox had been eradicated. There was a viewpoint, therefore, that all smallpox virus stored in laboratories throughout the world should be destroyed. That would prevent smallpox virus from escaping if there were a laboratory accident. However, smallpox virus has been maintained in freezers in a number of laboratories, because countries were concerned that others might surreptitiously keep viable virus. There was concern that if one country kept viable virus, opportunities for biological warfare by that country would exist.

Vaccines in the past usually consisted of killed or weakened virus. More recently, vaccines have been made that consist of only the proteins of the virus or only viral mRNA, which leads to the viral proteins being made in the recipient (to which B cells then make antibody). Since virus is not administered, infection by the virus is not possible. See Table 4.1 for antiviral vaccines and Table 4.2 for SARS-CoV-2 vaccines. RNA vaccines are discussed below.

The goal for vaccines is active immunization that will be long lasting. This need be separated from passive immunization, whereby IgG (polyclonal or monoclonal) is administered. Passive immunization by the intravenous administration of IgG can be effective but is short lasting.

Table 4.1 Commonly used antiviral vaccines	
Virus	**Formulation of the vaccine**
Rabies	Inactivated (killed virus)*
Poliomyelitis	Inactivated**
Measles	Attenuated (weakened virus)***
Mumps	Attenuated
Rubella	Attenuated
Influenza	Inactivated (given by injection) and attenuated (given by nasal spray)
Papilloma	Subunit (protein from the virus)
Varicella (chickenpox)	Attenuated
Shingles (herpes zoster)	Recombinant subunit****
Hepatitis A	Inactivated
Hepatitis B	Subunit

Table 4.1 (cont.)

Virus	Formulation of the vaccine
Rotavirus	Attenuated
Smallpox	Animal virus***** (cowpox virus vaccine)

[*] People exposed to rabies virus also receive anti-rabies IgG (passive immunization) against the rabies virus.

[**] Oral polio virus (attenuated) had been used widely in the past and is still used in some places. It probably produces superior immunity, but rare cases of clinical polio were noted, 2–4 cases per million doses.

[***] Measles vaccine is often administered along with mumps and rubella vaccines as MMR vaccine.

[****] An older vaccine used the same attenuated virus preparation as for childhood varicella immunization, but at a higher dose. Varicella and shingles are caused by the same virus. This vaccine is being discontinued for adults. More recent is a protein recombinant shingles vaccine.

[*****] Cowpox virus, related to human smallpox virus, was developed and widely used prior to the elimination of clinical smallpox.

Table 4.2 SARS-CoV-2 vaccines being made in Western Europe and the United States

Company	Formulation of the vaccine
Moderna*	Viral spike protein mRNA (mRNA-1273)
Pfizer-BioNTech*	Viral spike protein mRNA (BNT162b2)
CureVac-GSK*	Viral spike protein mRNA (CVnCoV)
Johnson & Johnson**	Replication incompetent adenovirus encoding viral spike protein (Ad26.CoV.S)
AstraZeneca/Oxford**	Replication incompetent adenovirus encoding viral spike protein (AZS1222)
Novavax ***	Viral spike protein (NVX-CoV2373)
Sanofi-GSK***	Viral spike protein (VAT00008)

[*] Viral mRNA with a lipid nanoparticle coat.

[**] Viral mRNA in a harmless (noncoronavirus) virus.

[***] Subunit vaccine, immunizing with viral spike protein.

Much is being learned about the immune response to SARS-CoV-2 and to other coronaviruses and will likely have significant clinical impact. It has been noted that some people who had been infected with SARS-CoV (to be differentiated from SARS-CoV-2) in 2003 have antibody to SARS-CoV-2. Also, some with antibody to SARS-CoV-2 have antibody reactivity to SARS-CoV and Middle East respiratory syndrome (MERS).

As noted in Chapter 1, the coronaviruses that caused the illnesses SARS, MERS, and COVID-19, along with two coronaviruses that cause the common cold, are members of the beta corona virus genus. Some overlap of immune reactivity among the viruses might be expected to occur. The goals in terms of SARS-CoV-2 vaccine development are vaccines that are effective against multiple variants, and immunoreactivity to other coronaviruses may be important in that regard.

Generally speaking, live virus vaccines may produce a slightly better antibody response than a comparable killed or subunit vaccine, but there is a slight risk of overt infection with the former. As noted in Table 4.1, live attenuated poliomyelitis virus vaccine has been supplanted in much of the world by the use of killed virus vaccine, because the former occasionally caused clinical polio. The frequency has been estimated to be about two to four cases of clinical polio in a million live virus vaccine recipients. In an example such as this, it would be important to know the degree to which the different vaccines protect against clinical polio.

The development of the poliomyelitis virus vaccine was one of the triumphs of twentieth-century science/medicine. Jonas Salk developed the injectable inactivated vaccine most widely used today, and some have wondered why he did not receive a Nobel Prize. The Nobel Prize in Physiology/Medicine was awarded in 1954 to John Enders, Frederick Robbins, and Thomas Weller, who in 1949 discovered methods to grow the poliomyelitis virus in cell culture – methods that permitted the development of the polio vaccine. Enders later developed the measles virus vaccine in 1960. Oral attenuated poliomyelitis vaccines were developed by Hilary Koprowski and Albert Sabin.

TOXOID VACCINES

Toxoid **vaccines**, although not antiviral vaccines, because of the important and interesting concept, are briefly mentioned here. Human vaccines against tetanus toxin and against diphtheria toxin – toxoid vaccines – are very effective. In both instances, the bacterial toxins are used to actively immunize people against the bacterial toxins, and not to immunize them against the bacteria. Similarly, toxins such as rattlesnake venom (a toxin) can be used to make a vaccine (a toxoid vaccine) against rattlesnake venom. The administration of these vaccines results in active immunization.

Toxoid vaccines produce an immune response against a toxic protein, and one could speculate on the development of such vaccines for various illnesses. For example, monoclonal antibodies against a specific cellular protein are being developed to treat patients with Alzheimer's disease. Might an mRNA vaccine specifically directed against that protein be useful?

Interestingly, a toxoid vaccine was used to treat people before there was knowledge of Ig and antibody. And people were passively (not actively) immunized. People at risk for diphtheria received serum from horses that had been immunized with diphtheria toxin, since it appeared that there was a "protective factor" in the blood of such horses. The horses had been immunized with diphtheria toxin; that is, they received a toxoid vaccine. Horse serum was administered to people containing the protective factor – passive immunization. Emil von Behring was awarded the Nobel Prize in Physiology/Medicine in 1901 (the first Nobel in Physiology/Medicine) for that treatment of individuals with diphtheria.

CLINICAL VACCINE ISSUES

The SARS-CoV-2 vaccines have clearly been effective.[38–41]

However, as is the case for new medications, questions, particularly in terms of possible side effects, have come up. As is the case for all medical treatments, the risk : benefit ratio is the crux of the issue. For the SARS-CoV-2 vaccines, the benefits greatly outweigh the risks.

The following section focuses on vaccines for COVID-19, although similar points can be considered for all vaccines.

Pregnancy

Multiple issues are of routine concern by clinicians when considering vaccine immunization, and many of these have been brought to the fore by the COVID-19 pandemic. Caution might be considered in situations such as pregnancy where relatively few pregnant women have been followed in SARS-CoV-2 immunization studies. However, in part since there is no live virus in any of the commonly used vaccines, it appears that SARS-CoV-2 immunization is safe for pregnant woman and their fetuses Newborns have been normal, and antibody has been detected in their blood. Antibody has also been detected in the milk of lactating mothers. Newborns with antibody that crossed over to them from the placenta during pregnancy or who received antibody in their mothers' milk have been passively immunized, and they will lose such antibody, with a half-life of about 1 month.

Fertility

There has been no evidence of any of the vaccines resulting in impaired fertility. This has been more directly studied in men, where sperm were directly studied. From semen analysis before and after SARS-CoV-2 vaccine administration, there was no decrease in the number of motile sperm.[41] There has also been no evidence that pregnancies were terminated by vaccines or that there was increased rate of miscarriage.

Immunosuppressed Patients

People who are immunosuppressed because of illness or because of medications they have been receiving have two issues in terms of vaccine immunization: (1) Is the vaccine safe? (2) Will the vaccine result in an appropriate immune response? In terms of the issue of safety, it is likely that RNA SARS-CoV-2 vaccines are safe, since live virus is not present, and therefore, virus cannot infect the individual.

First, use of live virus vaccines is generally a concern in immunosuppressed individuals. Concern is that the virus in the vaccine might replicate and cause illness since the individual's immune system is impaired. In some situations, it has been common for patients who are to receive immunosuppression medication to receive live viral vaccine several weeks before they start immunosuppression, to avoid giving live virus to immunosuppressed individuals.

Second, there is concern that immunosuppression may diminish the immune response to the vaccine, for example, the antibody response to a SARS-CoV-2 vaccine. Immunization in immunosuppressed individuals has been noted to result in lower antibody titers than in nonimmunosuppressed individuals. For that reason, some immunosuppressed individuals may require more frequent vaccine administration than do those who are not immunosuppressed.

Monoclonal antibody treatment, including repeated treatment, may be of value in preventing development of illness in those who are immunosuppressed.

Can People Who Are SARS-CoV-2 Immunized Be Infected by SARS-CoV-2?

First, it is well known that immunization in general does not prevent infection and illness in all people. This is probably in part related to the degree of the immune response of individuals, including antibody and T cell responses.

Second, while in some instances immunization has appeared to prevent clinical illness, it has not prevented subsequent detection of virus, for example, PCR detection of SARS-CoV-2 RNA in nasopharyngeal swabs. As discussed in Chapter 1, this RNA probably does indicate the presence of infectious virus. However, the amount of virus is likely lesser than in the nonimmunized.

We can consider these immunized but virus-positive individuals in terms of differences between epidemiology and clinical medicine.

As discussed in Chapter 1, in the past people with no symptoms would not usually have been tested for the presence of viral nucleic acid. It would not be a clinical concern – the individuals were doing well and most clinicians would likely not have tested such asymptomatic individuals. Largely epidemiological concerns, including following paths of infection in others, led to their being tested.

Leaving aside epidemiological issues, it would seem that positive PCR SARS-CoV-2 results from throat swabs of previously immunized individuals support the value of immunization – because these individuals have usually not been sick. Despite the presence of virus in their throat swabs, they were asymptomatic, and it can be considered that immunization prevented them from being sick.

Viral Variants

As discussed in Chapter 1, in considering the occurrence of influenza virus that may change year to year, resulting in decreased effectiveness of vaccines, a key issue in discussing SARS-CoV-2 variants is probably whether current vaccines are effective. A variant might be more transmissible or might cause more severe illness, but the main clinical question would likely be whether the variant is recognized by and thereby inhibited by current vaccines.

While early in the story, thus far it seems that variants are recognized and inhibited by the current vaccines. If not, the alternative would be creating new vaccines, as is done almost yearly for influenza virus vaccines. The development of RNA vaccines would likely make this a simpler and quicker process than has been the case in the past. It would not be a surprise if in the future people received SARS-CoV-2 booster shots, possibly with a vaccine other than the one they initially received. As this is being written, there is much discussion of "mixing and matching," that is, administering a SARS-CoV-2 vaccine other than that initially administered as a "booster."

Viral variants are very common and are the rule rather than the exception in clinical virology.

Vaccine Side Effects

Vaccine development has been a real triumph in science/medicine and has saved very many lives. Side effects are modest but can occur. For example, some vaccines produce fever, and infants are at risk for febrile seizures; seizures of this type can occur with any cause of fever. Important to note: febrile seizures in infants do not increase the risk of seizures later in life. People with multiple allergies have a greater risk of severe allergic reactions after receiving vaccines.

There is no evidence that COVID-19 or other vaccines cause autism.

In terms of people receiving one of the COVID-19 vaccines, most side effects have been mild and short lasting, including injection site pain, mild fever, and headache. Some people have had side effects more so after the first dose of two-shot vaccines and some after the second.

Severe vaccine side effects have been uncommon, including anaphylaxis after receiving COVID-19 vaccines. Anaphylaxis, a severe acute allergic condition that may require breathing support, has been noted in about five individuals per million doses of vaccine. Occurrence of anaphylaxis was more frequent in women and occurred usually within several minutes of immunization. Many anaphylaxis patients had a history of multiple allergies and had a history of prior anaphylaxis.[42,43]

Most patients who developed anaphylaxis did not require breathing support. And most patients did well after the treatment of anaphylaxis.

An important but uncommon side effect noted after administration of the Moderna and Pfizer vaccines has been myocarditis (inflammation of the heart muscle) and pericarditis (inflammation of the membrane around the heart).[44] This occurred primarily in men with a frequency of 25 to 30 per million doses of vaccine. Patients did well after supportive treatment.

A potentially more severe but less common complication, noted rarely after receiving the single dose vaccines (Johnson & Johnson and AstraZeneca) was venous thrombosis, particularly cerebral venous thrombosis.[45] As is true for many cases of venous thrombosis throughout the body, edema and hemorrhage may occur. This is often more significant when it involves the brain than other sites of thrombosis. Almost all cases of venous sinus thrombosis have been in women, and an autoimmune connection seems likely. Autoantibodies in these rare patients have been noted, similar to those in rare patients with a similar thrombosis syndrome after receiving heparin medication.

The issue of potential immune-mediated vaccine side effects (vaccines in general), for example, Guillain-Barré syndrome, is further discussed in Chapter 7.

It is very likely that with the further development of mRNA vaccines, the issue of vaccine side effects will be decreased.

RNA Vaccines

Vaccines depend on viral proteins triggering an immune response to the proteins. That is, B and T cells recognize a viral protein – or part of a viral protein, the epitope. The viral protein recognized may be part of live (attenuated) or killed virus, purified viral protein, or more recently viral protein produced in the vaccine recipient after the administration of viral mRNA.

As discussed in Chapter 3, mRNA is translated into protein, and with viral mRNA vaccines, viral protein antigen is made in the recipient. There is no virus present. The mRNA translation to protein occurs in the cell cytoplasm, and so the mRNA does not come into contact with cell DNA.

The process is new, and so varied methods are being used to determine the best response. People have used pure mRNA, but this may be at the mercy of ribonucleases, which we all have in our bodies and which degrade RNA. Therefore, laboratories have utilized methods to try to protect the mRNA from degradation by the use of coatings of different types, as well as other methods. It is too early to say which of the processes to protect the RNA in future vaccines will be shown to be the best.

It is very likely that mRNA vaccines will be widely used in the future. Such vaccines against SARS-CoV-2 are likely the beginning of other RNA vaccines. RNA vaccines are more like pharmaceuticals, medications that have been developed to treat illnesses and symptoms of illnesses, than they are like biologics, including most previously available vaccines. The future of RNA vaccines is wide open. It is possible to speculate that if RNAs can be isolated from other than viral illnesses, they could be used to prevent/treat those other illnesses.

Further Reading

AK Abbas, AH Lichtman, S Pillai. *Cellular and Molecular Immunology*, 10th ed. Elsevier Health Sciences, 2017

F Bagnoli, R Rappuoli. *Advanced Vaccine Research: Methods for the Decade of Vaccines*, Caister Academic Press, 2015. Book 978–1–91090–03–6 E-book 978–1–91090–04–3

5

Viral Pathogenesis

Viral pathogenesis refers to the mechanisms by which viral infections cause disease. Important are the cell types that viruses infect, virus replication in those cells, and host mechanisms of resistance such as immune reactivity.

In terms of the pathogenesis of nervous system infections, viruses usually enter the nervous system subsequent to viremia (virus from the bloodstream enters the nervous system) – poliomyelitis virus, arboviruses, or by neural axoplasmic transport (rabies, herpes simplex virus, varicella-zoster virus). Axonal transport is discussed below.

Lytic and Latent Virus Infections

Pathogenesis, the disease progression caused by a virus, very much depends on the virus being considered. Important are the molecular biological mechanisms by which the virus replicates after entering a cell. Several types of viral infections can be considered.

An active, lytic infection is one in which infectious virus invades susceptible cells and in which infectious virus rapidly replicates. A lytic infection denotes lysis, the destruction of infected cells. This is the type of virus infection most people consider when they discuss viral infections. The entire viral genome is replicated and viral-specified DNAs, RNAs, and proteins are present.

A chronic or persistent infection is similar to this type of infection, but the infection occurs at a low level, possibly because the host immune system keeps the infection under some control. Viral DNAs, RNAs, and proteins are present, albeit possibly in small amounts. A persistent infection would be quantitatively different from a lytic infection but probably not qualitatively different.

In latent infections, however, the infection is qualitatively different from lytic infections. Latent virus infections are different in that while the entire viral genome is present, replication of the genome does not occur, and expression of viral DNAs, RNAs, and proteins is very limited. In latent herpesvirus infections, for example, the viral DNA is thought to be present in latently infected cells as an episome, separate from the cellular DNA. On occasion, latent viral infections undergo reactivation, at which time viral genome replication occurs and viral RNAs and proteins are expressed.

A slow virus infection, such as subacute sclerosing panencephalitis (a type of measles virus infection), may be thought of as a low-level persistent infection, and progressive multifocal leukoencephalopathy (JC virus infection) as the result of a latent viral infection that has reactivated. Both are discussed in Chapter 7.

The term "lysogeny" (lysogenic infection) describes a type of infection of bacteria by bacteriophage, with the integration of the bacteriophage DNA into that of the bacteria – the virus and the bacterial cell replicate together. This type of infection led to early considerations of how, if viral DNA integrated into cellular DNA, viruses might cause cancer.

In part, definitions of viral latency rely on the absence of specific viral gene products during latency. It is always important to consider whether the inability to detect these products is due to their absence or simply the lack of methods sensitive enough to detect them. In some ways, relying on the absence of viral RNAs and proteins to define latency is in the category of trying to prove a negative – that is, trying to prove that they are not present.

As part of many investigations, the concepts of latent viral infections developed, with emphasis on the human herpesviruses, all of which establish latent infections.[46] Latent infections have been best studied for HSV and Epstein–Barr virus (EBV). Human immunodeficiency virus (HIV) and the related human T-lymphotropic virus type 1 also establish latent infections. Human BK and JC polyoma viruses probably establish latent infections.

In this volume, emphasis is placed on viruses known to cause infections of the nervous system. Examples include rabies virus, poliomyelitis virus, and arboviruses, all of which cause acute lytic infections. Human immunodeficiency virus, herpes simplex virus, and varicella-zoster virus cause both lytic and latent types of infections.

Viral Latency vs the Latent Period of an Infection

Before leaving this introduction to viral latency, differentiating it from the latent period of a viral infection need be mentioned.

After virus exposure/infection, there is a period early in the infection process, called the latent period, before which clinical symptoms are not yet apparent. However, a better term than "latent period" prior to the onset of symptoms is "incubation period." This might be the time between a mosquito bite and the start of clinical symptoms.

The occurrence of an incubation period before symptoms are recognized by a virus-infected individual is common for many virus infections. During this incubation period, virus may replicate, and some cells may be destroyed (lytic infection), but the individual is not yet clinically aware of the infection. This might be the time between a nasopharyngeal SARS-CoV-2-positive polymerase chain reaction (PCR) result and the onset of clinical symptoms.

The occasional use of the term "latent period" for such a prelude to an overt clinical infection is unrelated to the concept of viral latency.

SARS-CoV-2

Although emphasis here is on viral infections of the nervous system, because of their contemporary importance, discussion of viral pathogenesis begins with the pathogenesis of three viruses where viral infection of the nervous system occurs but is not paramount.

The pathogenesis of SARS-CoV-2 infection, the illness commonly known as COVID-19, is being sorted out at present. It is apparent that respiratory involvement is paramount. The innate and adaptive immune responses of most patients act to control the infection,[32,33] with those who have other underlying illnesses or are of advanced age most at risk for more severe and possibly lethal infections. Overall mortality is ~2%. In some patients, there may be overreactivity of the innate immune system with "cytokine storm" resulting, and this inflammation may cause significant morbidity.[34,47]

While inflammation has been detected in the brains of COVID-19 patients who died with the illness, viral RNA has not.[48]

The COVID-19 pandemic has likely altered the care of patients in several ways. First is the emphasis on its epidemiology (Chapter 1), the pathways by which virus is transmitted from person to person. Related to this is the emphasis on PCR testing, which is likely to greatly expand in considering other infectious illnesses. Many people are now aware of transmission of viruses such as SARS-CoV-2 by the respiratory route.

Second, much recent emphasis has been on vaccine development to prevent illness. Vaccine use (Chapter 4) is important in preventing infection.[38–40]

In terms of other treatments to minimize infection that has occurred, monoclonal and polyclonal antibodies (Chapter 4) may be useful, as may antiviral medications (Chapter 3).

Viral infection per se may cause damage to organ systems, and in some individuals after a viral infection, autoimmune neurological illnesses such as Guillain-Barré syndrome may occur (Chapter 7). In terms of specific neurological symptoms with COVID-19, the most common has been anosmia, the loss of the sense of smell, usually for 3 to 8 weeks.

It has been noted that there may be late symptoms in some individuals after the viral infection has seemingly cleared. Symptoms in these individuals are variable and include fatigue, shortness of breath, cough, joint pain, chest pain, difficulty concentrating, depression, muscle pain, and headache. Interestingly, there has not been a clear relationship between the severity of the COVID-19 illness and such symptoms. People with these symptoms have been termed as having COVID long-hauler syndrome, long COVID syndrome, and post-COVID syndrome.

In some ways, long COVID syndrome seems similar to the chronic fatigue syndrome attributed by some to Epstein–Barr virus infection. A direct viral or other cause (for example, inflammatory illness) and the treatment of long COVID syndrome remain to be determined.

Human Immunodeficiency Virus (HIV)

Before SARS-CoV-2, the virus that led to much recent interest and growth in virology was human immunodeficiency virus (HIV). HIV type 1 (HIV-1) and the slightly less virulent HIV-2 may cause the acquired immunodeficiency disease syndrome (AIDS). Françoise Barré-Sinoussi and Luc Montagnier won the Nobel Prize in Physiology/Medicine in 2008 for their discovery of HIV as the cause of AIDS.

HIV is thought to enter the body through oral or genital mucous membranes. From initial sites of entry, HIV typically is brought to lymph nodes by macrophages or other similar cells, termed "dendritic cells." Macrophages and dendritic cells often bind foreign material and bring it to lymph nodes, where an immune response to the agent may be initiated.

HIV brought to lymph nodes infects multiple cell types of the nodes, most notably CD 4 T lymphocytes (Chapter 4). Virus is replicated, and viremia often results; virus enters the bloodstream and passes throughout the body.

Innate immune factors including interferons are produced by multiple cell types in an attempt to limit the viral infection. Subsequently, aspects of the adaptive immune response such as antibody production are brought to bear, and the HIV infection is limited. However, it is not completely cleared. It is not eliminated from susceptible CD 4 T lymphocytes.

Over time, the degree of HIV infection may be followed by the measurement of amounts of virus in the bloodstream (the viral load) and by the measurement of number of remaining/surviving CD 4 T lymphocytes. If/when CD 4 cells are depleted, the immune response to many antigens may be impaired. If the CD 4 T cell depletion is severe, the infected individual may develop clinical AIDS.

The CD 4 T lymphocytes are often considered as "helper" T cells and are important for aspects of the immune response to multiple pathogens (Chapter 4). The depletion of CD 4 T cells may result in varied infections. Discussion of one, progressive multifocal leukoencephalopathy (PML), caused by the JC polyoma virus, is presented in Chapter 7.

In some CD 4 T lymphocytes, the HIV virus (an RNA virus) enters a latent state. In these cells, the virus exists as a DNA provirus (a DNA copy of the viral RNA), which is incorporated into the cellular DNA. At that time, virus is not synthesized in the cell, and infection of the cell is not readily apparent. Subsequently, reactivation from latency with the production of infectious virus may occur. This reactivated virus may infect new CD 4 T lymphocytes and thereby continue the HIV infection. Virus may be transmitted to other people.

Multiple antiviral medications have been shown to have significant impacts on limiting virus replication. Azidothymidine (AZT) (zidovudine [ZDA]) was the first effective HIV antiviral (Chapter 3), and more than

20 others have been approved. Recently, emphasis has been on the use of combinations of medications. Combinations decrease the problem of viral resistance that may occur to a single medication. Most recent are viral integrase inhibitors. While the medications are useful in decreasing virus load in infected individuals, during HIV latent infection there is no apparent viral synthetic biochemical machinery present, and so no clear target for antiviral medications.[49,50]

Similarly, during latency there is no viral antigen target for antiviral antibody. For these reasons, HIV is not be eliminated from the individual. While antibody is effective in decreasing HIV during the period of acute infection, it does not eliminate the latent virus infection. Methods to identify latently infected lymphocytes, a possible forerunner to eliminating them by novel HIV vaccine developments, continues.

HIV can be maintained in a latent state as a DNA provirus in latently infected CD 4 lymphocytes for years. One could speculate on the possibility that in the presence of antiviral medications and continued intermittent reactivation, the pool of latently infected cells might eventually become depleted.

In rare instances, a few individuals seem to have cleared the virus, and it would be of great importance to determine possible mechanisms. First, the observation would need to be verified, and this is not as easy as might seem. It raises the difficult issue of proving a negative. How many and what types of tests would need show no evidence of HIV to "prove" the individual has cleared the virus?

As noted in Chapter 6, HIV infection may cause a viral meningitis, typically early in the course of infection. Prior to the availability of effective antivirals, neurological involvement of HIV-infected individuals was common, including encephalopathy (AIDS dementia complex), severe neuropathy, and spinal cord impairment (vacuolar myelopathy).

Impaired immunity led to intercurrent viral infections, particularly cytomegalovirus and JC virus (human polyoma virus, Chapter 7), infections of the nervous system. AIDS-related EBV infection led to lymphoproliferative illnesses and lymphomas. Multiple types of infections and neoplasms caused severe illness and death prior to the availability of effective antivirals.

Epstein–Barr Virus (EBV)

The currently known human herpesviruses include herpes simplex virus-type 1 (HSV-1), HSV-2, varicella-zoster virus (VZV), cytomegalovirus (CVM), Epstein–Barr virus (EBV), human herpesvirus-6 (HHV-6), human herpesvirus-7 (HHV-7), and human herpesvirus-8 (HHV-8).

HSV-1 is known to cause "cold sores" of the face and may infect the eyes. Occasionally it may cause more systemic infection including meningitis and encephalitis (Chapters 6, 7). HSV-2 is known as a cause of recurrent genital infections. VZV is the cause of chickenpox in children and herpes zoster (shingles) in adults. CMV may cause birth defects, and it may cause a mononucleosis-like illness. EBV is the usual cause of "mono" (infectious mononucleosis) and has been associated with some cancers. HHV-6 and HHV-7 may cause skin rash and fever in children, and HHV-8 has been associated with Kaposi sarcoma.

There are also many animal herpesviruses, most of which do not infect humans – but see human infection by herpes B virus of macaque monkeys (Chapter 6).

The alpha human herpesviruses that establish latent infections in neurons include HSV-1, HSV-2, and VZV. The beta human herpesviruses include cytomegalovirus, HHV-6, and HHV-7. The gamma human herpesviruses that establish latent infections of lymphocytes include EBV and HHV-8.

Epstein–Barr virus is transmitted by saliva and is the most common cause of human mononucleosis.[51] At the time of initial infection, epithelial cells are infected and produce infectious virus. These cells undergo lytic infections. B lymphocytes (Chapter 4) are subsequently infected and may undergo long-term latent infection. It is likely that 90% or more of people are latently infected with EBV.

Infectious virus and all of the complete panoply of viral RNAs and proteins are not present during latency.

Much complexity exists during EBV latency, including three latency types (I, II, III), each with limited and distinct viral RNAs and proteins being expressed. During latent infection, the EBV DNA genome is in a circular episomal form and is not integrated into the cellular DNA.[46] The human latent B lymphocyte infection is lifelong. At times during latency, reactivation may occur in B lymphocytes; the circular viral DNA takes a linear form and infectious virus is produced.

Part of the great interest in EBV relates to it causing Burkitt lymphoma and possibly other neoplasms. Burkitt was a physician who described the unique lymphoma that bears his name. Epstein and Barr discovered virus particles in the tumor cells, subsequently named Epstein–Barr virus (EBV).

In addition to being the cause of Burkitt lymphoma, EBV has been associated with nasopharyngeal cancer, gastric cancer, and Hodgkin lymphoma. Specifics insofar as mechanisms of EBV long-term latency, reactivation, and mechanisms by which cancers occur remain to be determined. There has been much interest as well of EBV playing a role in the neurological illness multiple sclerosis (Chapter 7).

EBV has occasionally been associated with illnesses of the nervous system, such as encephalitis. A difficulty has been in determining whether the virus caused an infection of brain cells, or if it caused an immune inflammatory reaction that damaged brain cells. The latter immunologically mediated illness is often called acute disseminated encephalomyelitis (ADEM). Such immunologically mediated illnesses (post-infectious or para-infectious) are often a clinical issue (Chapter 7).

EBV vaccines are currently in the early stages of development. Goals will likely be the treatment of patients with neoplasms where EBV has been implicated, but treatment of other illnesses, such as chronic fatigue syndrome, may also be a target. This illness is somewhat ill defined but has often been related to EBV infection. As noted above, the long COVID syndrome has similarities to chronic fatigue syndrome. EBV vaccines have also been discussed by some as a possible means to prevent illness such as mononucleosis and, theoretically at this time, to prevent multiple sclerosis (Chapter 7).

Specific mRNA vaccines to EBV proteins may provide a means to approach eliminating latent EBV infections.

Herpes Simplex Virus (HSV)

In this section, viral infections of the nervous system start with discussion of HSV, a common infection of neurons.

Recurrent cold sores and recurrent genital infection by HSV-1 and HSV-2, respectively, are clinical hallmarks of these herpesviruses; after an initial oral or genital infection, a latent infection in neurons is established, and when HSV-1 and HSV-2 reactivate from the latent infection, recurrent clinical infection results – cold sores, genital infection.

HSV latent infections are established in sensory ganglion neurons, and with reactivation from latency, clinically apparent, lytic mucocutaneous infection may occur.

Importantly, in some people reactivation from latency and the production of infectious virus occur, but the individuals do not develop clinical illness or symptoms. They have the occurrence of asymptomatic virus shedding. One might hypothesize that they have no clinical symptoms because they have very low-level infections.

Similarly, after initial VZV skin infection (chickenpox), the virus may establish a latent infection in sensory ganglion neurons, and with reactivation in the future cause herpes zoster (shingles) – discussed below.

The initial cutaneous HSV or VZV infection is similar in many ways to other viral infections. Innate immunological factors are brought to bear by the host in an attempt to limit or eliminate the infection.

During the period of subsequent latent infection, adaptive immune factors are present, but, as discussed below, usually do not eliminate the latent infection. With reactivation, innate and adaptive immune factors limit the spread of the reactivated infection, but again they do not eliminate the continued latent infection.

The latent infections established by HSV and VZV are infections of neurons, and the basis of the recurrent infections they cause is viral reactivation in those latently infected neurons. Therefore, discussion of the pathogenesis of HSV-1, HSV-2, and VZV need include discussion of some aspects of neurobiology.

After an initial cutaneous clinical infection, HSV-1, HSV-2, and VZV travel by retrograde axoplasmic transport to the cell body and nucleus of sensory neurons in the trigeminal and dorsal root ganglia. Latent infections of these neurons develop.[46]

With reactivation of latent infection of trigeminal and dorsal root ganglion neurons, HSV and VZV travel from the latently infected neurons to the periphery, the skin and mucous membranes, by orthograde axoplasmic transport. At skin and mucous membrane sites, clinically apparent infections may be seen.[52]

The neurons of the trigeminal and dorsal root ganglia do not replicate, and so the ganglion neurons individuals are born with are the neurons they have for their lives. It is thought teleologically that HSV and VZV are well adapted to their existence in these lifelong cells as a means to permit very long-term infection. Features of latent infection and reactivation in these neurons are discussed below.

After early, probably childhood infection by HSV, lifelong latent infection may result, even in people who do not have a history of cold sores. This has led to the herpes virology joke: What is the difference between HSV and love? – HSV is forever.

Trigeminal and Dorsal Root Ganglion Neurons

Neurons in which these latent infections are established are neurons of the trigeminal and dorsal root ganglia. Humans have two trigeminal ganglia, right and left; they mediate sensation from the face, eyes, mouth, and head. The dorsal root ganglia are smaller but more numerous; humans have 62 of them (31 pairs on the right and 31 pairs on the left). They medicate sensation from the rest of the body.

These sensory ganglia are composed of large neurons, with additional supporting cells and blood vessel cells. Although the neurons are larger than other cells throughout the body, some ganglion neurons are larger than are others, and their functions are likely different.

The following discussion focuses on the trigeminal system (Fig. 5.1), but information presented can be directly applied to the very similar dorsal root ganglion system.

The trigeminal ganglion is a cluster of sensory neurons (and non-neuron supporting cells) just below the brain and is not part of the brain. The ganglion is part of the peripheral nervous system. (The peripheral nervous system and the central nervous system are discussed in Chapter 7.)

As shown in Figure 5.1, there is a distal projection of each ganglion neuron to the skin of the face and the eyes (the trigeminal nerve), and a proximal projection of each neuron (the trigeminal root) to the brain. When the face is touched, sensation is perceived because the trigeminal nerve is stimulated. The stimulus alters function of the nerve, and impulses pass up the nerve, to the ganglion neurons and then via the trigeminal root to the brain. The neurons in the trigeminal ganglia are sensory neurons.

The cell bodies of motor neurons (not shown in Fig. 5.1) are in the spinal cord and parts of the brainstem. Their axons extend to muscle cells and control the contraction of muscles and resulting movement.

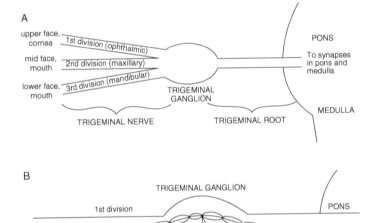

Figure 5.1 A. Diagram of the trigeminal system: trigeminal ganglion, trigeminal nerve, trigeminal root. It includes three branches of the nerve that extend distally to different parts of the face and head, the trigeminal ganglion, and the trigeminal root that extends proximally from the ganglion to the brain (the pons and medulla are lower parts of the brain). B. Detail of one branch of the nerve showing an individual ganglion neuron and axon. The tubular axon is a continuation of the cell – the axoplasm in an axon is continuous with the neuronal cytoplasm.

Axons are covered with electrical insulating myelin (except very distally). The myelin, which covers axons just outside of and inside the brain (the medulla, pons in Fig. 5.1), is made by oligodendrocytes. The myelin over the remaining parts of the axon is made by Schwann cells. The "two myelins" are chemically different, and different illnesses may result from damage (demyelination) to them. Multiple sclerosis results from oligodendrocyte demyelination and Guillain-Barré syndrome from Schwann cell demyelination. Discussion of these illnesses is presented in Chapter 7.

Axoplasmic Transport

Axons are an extension of neurons, and the axoplasm is a continuation of the neuronal cytoplasm. Strikingly, the axoplasm is not quiescent but contains active processes. Both anterograde and retrograde axoplasmic transport occur, albeit at different rates. Anterograde transport is from the neuronal cell body to the periphery, for example, to the face. Retrograde transport is from the periphery (the face) to the neuronal cell body.

HSV and VZV use retrograde axoplasmic transport to pass from peripheral sites of initial cutaneous or mucous membrane infection to neurons that become latently infected. And they use anterograde transport to pass from sites of reactivation in latently infected ganglion neurons to the periphery, where overt skin and mucous membrane infection may be manifested.[52]

AXOPLASMIC TRANSPORT IN OTHER HUMAN DISEASES

Axoplasmic transport is important in considering the pathogenesis of two bacterial infections – botulism and tetanus. Botulism is caused by the toxin of *Clostridia* (*Clostridioides*) *botulinum* and tetanus by the toxin of *Clostridia* (*Clostridioides*) *tetani*. The bacteria are similar and the toxins are similar – both inhibit neurotransmitter release – but the illnesses are very dissimilar, in part because of axoplasmic transport.

The above discussion of HSV and VZV relates to sensory axons, which carry HSV from the skin to the trigeminal and dorsal root ganglia. Axons important for botulism and tetanus are motor axons that extend from the spinal cord motor neurons to muscles. Transmission of impulses via the axons of these neurons causes the contraction of muscles.

Botulinum toxin enters motor axons distally, at neuromuscular junctions. At that site, the most distal aspect of the motor axon, the toxin prevents the release of the neurotransmitter acetylcholine from the distal axon to the muscle cell.

Normally, acetylcholine passes from distal axons to muscle cells and causes electrical changes in the muscle cells, which results in muscle contraction. Botulinum toxin prevents the release of acetylcholine. Muscle weakness and, when severe, paralysis of muscle activity result. In the contemporary world, botulinum toxin is used by some to paralyze facial muscles, and thereby to eliminate facial wrinkles.

Tetanus toxin similarly enters motor axons distally, at the neuromuscular junction. However, this toxin is transported by retrograde axoplasmic flow to the cell bodies of motor neurons. It then passes proximally to adjacent neurons in the spinal cord. In those adjacent neurons, tetanus toxin also inhibits the release of neurotransmitter. However, that neurotransmitter, gamma-aminobutyric acid (GABA), is an inhibitory transmitter. Inhibition of the inhibitory transmitter results in muscles continuously contracting, with muscle spasm occurring. When severe, muscles may go into spasm, including muscles for breathing.

RABIES

In terms of viral infections where axoplasmic transport is important, rabies virus infection has been well described. Rabies virus infection of humans, fortunately rare, is often a lethal infection of the brain. In keeping with the preceding discussion of axoplasmic transport, rabies virus is thought to pass to the brain by axoplasmic transport.

From the site of a bite by a rabid animal, transport of the virus to the brain occurs by that axoplasmic transport. Virus spreads proximally, up motor axons (as does tetanus toxin) and probably also up sensory axons (as do HSV and VZV). Virus then spreads in the brain. The infection is lethal unless patients are treated with rabies vaccine, and usually also with anti-rabies IgG in the form of rabies immune serum (Chapter 6).

HSV in the Trigeminal Ganglion

It has been known since the days of neurosurgeon Harvey Cushing, more than 100 years ago, that there is a relationship between HSV and the human trigeminal system (Fig. 5.1). When surgery was performed on the trigeminal system to treat the extremely severe pain of trigeminal neuralgia, HSV reactivation over the face was common.

Because of these observations, neurosurgeons removed part of the trigeminal ganglion (at the time of surgery for trigeminal neuralgia) and tested it for the presence of HSV, but HSV was not detected. These investigators homogenized ganglion tissue and cultured it on susceptible cells, the usual means to detect infectious virus, and the results were negative. Infectious virus was not detected. However, HSV was present in ganglion neurons in a latent state, as subsequently shown.

The fact that HSV is present and can be isolated from the trigeminal ganglia of experimental animals and of humans was demonstrated by Jack Stevens and Richard Barringer, respectively. They used explant culture techniques to permit the latent virus to reactivate, and thereby to be detected.

It is of interest that when random trigeminal ganglia were investigated at time of human autopsy (after various causes of death) and tested for HSV, latent virus was detected in many people, up to 90% in some studies – most of whom did not have histories of cold sores. It is likely that many/most of us have latent HSV infection of our trigeminal ganglia.

With explant techniques, it is thought that HSV reactivates in neurons that were latently infected and then replicates and infects other adjacent ganglion cells. The reactivation and replication of virus in the latently infected neurons requires the latently infected trigeminal ganglion neurons (which were obtained from dead individuals) to be "alive enough" to permit HSV to utilize cellular biochemical processes to reactivate.

An important point is that latent HSV (or latent VZV) infections are not simply low-grade infections, where the virus infection is slight. They are qualitatively different. HSV latent infection is not simply a low-grade infection by HSV, but rather it is a different type of infection. Experimental latent HSV infection is the emphasis of Chapter 8.

Criteria of Latent HSV Infection

During acute HSV infection (lytic infection), infectious virus, along with viral RNAs and proteins, is present. Infectious virus can be detected from swabs of skin lesions and can be similarly detected in homogenates of infected tissues or cells. Detection can be by the identification of HSV RNAs and proteins, and HSV can be readily grown and detected in cell culture.

However, these methods are not positive when latent HSV infection is present (with the exception of the detection of one viral RNA, discussed below), although infectious virus can be easily recovered by explant techniques.

An important marker of HSV latent infection is the presence of one specific viral RNA (transcribed from the viral DNA). The limited RNA present is discussed below as a hallmark of HSV latency. This viral RNA present during latency is called latency associated transcript (LAT). See Table 5.1 for criteria of types of HSV infections.

Studies over years by multiple investigators established the criteria of HSV latency, in human and experimental animal ganglia. During latency, the entire HSV DNA genome can be detected, but only one viral RNA, that is, LAT, is present.

Table 5.1 Criteria of types of HSV infections

	Lytic infection*	Latent infection
Infectious virus can be detected in infected tissue homogenates	Yes	No
Viral proteins (antigens) can be detected in infected tissue by immunological means	Yes	No
Complete viral DNA can be detected	Yes	Yes
Viral RNA can be detected		
Complete viral mRNAs	Yes	No
Only limited viral RNA (LAT)**	NA	Yes
Virus can be isolated by explant culture***	Yes	Yes

NA = not applicable.

* Initial acute infection and after reactivation.

** Specific HSV RNA termed latency associated transcript (LAT).

*** Explant culture of a tissue is performed by taking the tissue to be tested and culturing this tissue for several days in vitro. At that point, all HSV proteins, RNAs, and infectious virus are present.

Radiolabeled DNA probes were used to determine the presence of viral RNA; hybridization of DNA probes to complementary RNA targets was the goal.

Initial DNA probes to investigate HSV RNA present during latency consisted of fragments of the HSV DNA genome. These DNA fragments, prepared by cutting HSV genome DNA with restriction endonucleases, served as probes to detect HSV RNA that might be present. Using these methods, Jack Stevens showed that only very restricted HSV RNA was present in ganglion tissue, the LAT.

Subsequently, with knowledge of the deoxynucleotide sequence of the probe viral DNA fragment that was complementary to that RNA, it was possible to construct artificial deoxynucleotide sequences to search for (probe for) LAT.

In Situ Hybridization Detection of LAT RNA

As described in Chapter 3, an RNA and the DNA from which it is transcribed are complementary to each other. Therefore, DNA of specific sequence can be used as a probe to detect complementary RNA. For example, DNA of the hypothetical sequence dG-dG-dC-dG-dA-dT-dA-dA ... dC could be used to search for RNA of the sequence C-C-G-C-U-A-U-U ... G.

After being labeled, for example, with a radioactive isotope, and hybridization (binding) to the target RNA, the probe DNA would localize the presence of the target RNA. Such binding can be performed in blots of homogenized tissue (northern blot) or in in tissue sections (in situ hybridization).

The technique of in situ hybridization had been developed in part through the work of Harald zur Hausen, who won the Nobel Prize in Physiology/Medicine in 2008. He used in situ hybridization to detect human papillomavirus DNA in cervical carcinoma tissue. This led to the development of vaccines to decrease infection by this virus and to decrease cervical cancer risk.

To detect and determine the cellular localization of HSV LAT, a radioactive isotope was attached to a synthesized DNA probe consisting of a string of 20 deoxynucleotides. The radiolabeled DNA probe complementary to LAT RNA was placed on latently infected trigeminal ganglion tissue sections. After an appropriate length of time, the probe was removed. The tissue was washed and then overlaid with photographic emulsion. Again, after an appropriate length of time, the emulsion was developed, and areas where the radiolabeled probe had bound were detected (Fig. 5.2).

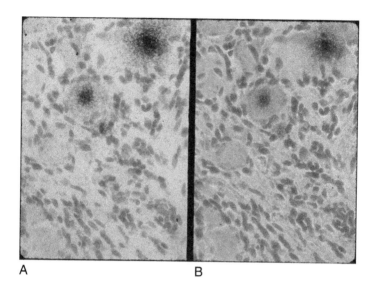

A B

Figure 5.2 In situ hybridization detection of HSV LAT RNA in neurons. A DNA probe labeled with radioactive isotope was placed on a tissue section of latently infected mouse trigeminal ganglion. After a period of time, the section was washed and overlaid with photographic emulsion. HSV RNA (LAT) in the tissue section is shown by the "grains" in the emulsion – where the DNA probe bound to target RNA. A. High-power magnification by standard light microscopy demonstrating two LAT-positive neurons. B. Label over the nuclei of the neurons is more clearly seen by phase contrast microscopy.

Subsequently, other labels such as biotin-labeled DNA probes were developed. These have been successfully used in place of radiolabeled probes. They give a colorimetric signal and avoid the issue of radioactivity.

The technique is termed "in situ hybridization" because hybridization is in situ, in tissue sections, rather than of a blot after homogenization and electrophoresis, as in a northern blot study. In either case, the DNA probe binds (hybridizes) to complementary target RNA. Studies in several laboratories showed that HSV LAT was present over the nucleus (and not other parts of the cell) of trigeminal ganglion neurons (Fig. 5.2) and (not over other cells).

HSV is a double-stranded DNA virus, and the viral DNA (the viral genome) codes for ~80 genes. Each DNA strand contains ~152,000 deoxynucleotides. However, HSV LAT RNA, which is transcribed from the viral DNA and expressed during latency, is only ~2,000 nucleotides long. Therefore, although the entire HSV DNA genome is present in ganglion neurons during latency, only ~1% of the genome is transcribed into viral RNA in latently infected neurons.

Interestingly, the HSV LAT RNA is not known to be translated to a viral protein. For that reason, in the preceding discussion, LAT has been termed an RNA rather than an mRNA. The role of LAT in HSV latency is unclear, but it is an established marker of HSV latency.

Thus far, it has not been possible to eliminate latent HSV infections, including by antibody to the virus, or through the use of the antiviral medication acyclovir (Chapter 8). The inability to eliminate the latent HSV infection through these means is similar to the inability to eliminate HIV latent infection (above).

Latent HSV Infection of the Brain?

As discussed above, there were historical reasons to suspect the trigeminal system (Fig. 5.1) as a possible site of HSV latency. The trigeminal ganglion neuron site was relatively easy to confirm, since the ganglia are relatively small and are easy to sample, or even investigate in their entirety.

There have been occasional suggestions that HSV may establish latent infections in other neurons, such as brain neurons. If that occurred, there would likely be discussions of possible illness that might result from the latent infection, and possible reactivation.

Preliminary studies of HSV latent infections of the brain of mice were performed. HSV was dropped into the nostrils of mice. It was expected that HSV would be transported to the brain by axoplasmic transport. Mice appeared normal. Four weeks later, the brains of these mice were examined by in situ hybridization to determine whether HSV latency was present. In these preliminary studies, the presence of HSV LAT was taken as evidence of HSV latency.

In Figure 5.3 are in situ hybridization results showing HSV LAT in brain neurons, neurons adjacent to the third ventricle of the brain.

There are four ventricles in the brain – two lateral ventricles (right and left), a third ventricle (midline), and a fourth ventricle (midline). Cerebrospinal fluid is produced in the ventricles – discussed in Chapter 7.

These results need be replicated and further investigated. It is possible to speculate on a possible role of latent HSV infection of the human brain and human HSV encephalitis (Chapter 6). Latent HSV infection of the brain might also be important to consider in other human illnesses. The pathogenesis of HSV latent infection of trigeminal ganglion neurons has been well described. Study of latent infection of brain neurons is a reasonable avenue for further investigation of HSV pathogenesis.

Experimental Animal Studies

Studies of HSV latent infection performed by the author and colleagues were performed with living adult mice. The latently infected living mice appeared to have normal behavior, and their eating, drinking, and weight were similar to that of uninfected mice. Study of trigeminal ganglion and brain tissues from these mice required them to be sacrificed (killed). Humane methods were used for this. In all instances, mice were anesthetized with sodium pentobarbital. When unconscious, cardiac puncture was performed, and blood was removed, resulting in death. Trigeminal ganglia (right and left) and brain tissues were then removed and studied for HSV latency.

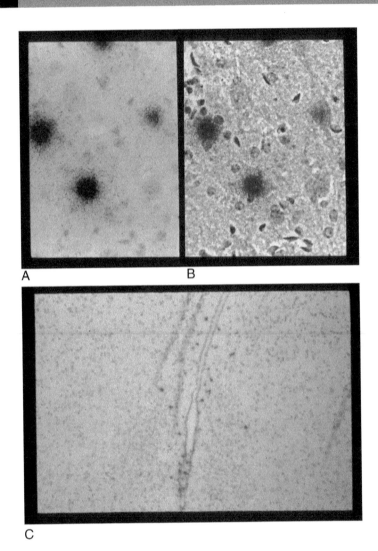

A   B

C

Figure 5.3 HSV LAT in mouse brain neurons, by in situ hybridization. A. Low-power photomicrograph showing LAT-positive, dark-labeled neurons on both sides of the vertical, slit-like third ventricle. B. High-power microscopy. C. High-power phase contrast microscopy showing LAT-positive neurons.

Therapeutic Deoxyribonucleotide Treatment (Antisense Inhibition)

The principle of hybridization of a specific deoxynucleotide (DNA) sequence to a specific RNA ribonucleotide target sequence (as above for in situ hybridization) has been discussed as a possible therapeutic modality. The plan would be to use a specific therapeutic DNA deoxynucleotide sequence to bind to an abnormal mRNA sequence in a patient.[53]

The goal would be for the therapeutic probe DNA to bind to specific target abnormal mRNA, and by that means inhibit its being translated into an abnormal protein. The probe DNA is antisense to the gene (Chapter 3) and so the process has been termed "antisense inhibition." The concept is further discussed in Chapter 9.

Varicella-Zoster Virus (VZV)

Varicella-**zoster virus** is very contagious in children, usually spreading by the airborne-respiratory route, by skin-to-skin contact, and through saliva. Initial infection is followed by blood-borne viremia and the development of blister-like pustules over the skin. Severe disseminated infection may occur, but not usually in immunocompetent individuals.

Skin vesicles contain live virus, which may travel to the nervous system by retrograde axoplasmic transport, as discussed above. VZV infection is subsequently maintained as a latent infection in sensory ganglion neurons (trigeminal or dorsal root). Much of the general picture of the establishment of HSV latency pertains to VZV latency.

With VZV reactivation, herpes zoster (shingles) is the usual clinical manifestation. Shingles typically occurs in the skin area subserved by neurons in one dorsal root or trigeminal ganglion. It is common for patients to note itch or pain in the area of skin that is destined to develop the vesicles of shingles a day or two later. This likely indicates that neurons in which reactivation has occurred are being stimulated.

Some have suggested the occurrence of similar symptoms of cutaneous itch and pain without evidence of shingles skin lesions as being due to zoster. Reactivation of VZV in ganglion neurons with cutaneous sensory symptoms but without skin lesions has been termed "zoster sine herpete."

Clinical zoster (shingles) severity is often related to immune status and age. Immunocompromised individuals are at risk for disseminated infection, and older individuals are at risk for severe pain, termed "post-herpetic neuralgia."

Antivirals of the class of acyclovir (Chapter 8) are commonly used to treat zoster, the reactivated infection. Immunization with VZV vaccines is commonly used to prevent the initial VZV infection in children and to decrease reactivated infection and zoster pain in adults.

A chickenpox vaccine first became available in 1995, with many children receiving it since then. The issues of duration of immune status and whether adults may develop clinical chickenpox as vaccine-related immunity wanes remain to be determined.

Initially, the same vaccine was used to prevent chickenpox in children and shingles in adults, although differing doses were used. More recently, a recombinant subunit vaccine has been used to prevent shingles in adults (Chapter 4).

Pain with VZV reactivation (zoster) is not uncommon and may occur at any age. However, long-lasting post-herpetic (post-shingles) pain is usually related to zoster in older individuals. It is often accompanied by patchy areas of decreased sensation around the areas of the skin that are painful.

Areas of decreased sensation after zoster might be due to the destruction of sensory ganglion neurons, in which viral reactivation had occurred. However, the concomitant occurrence of long-lasting pain suggests possible damage/destruction of brainstem and spinal cord neurons. These neurons receive connections from trigeminal ganglion and dorsal root ganglion neurons, respectively, and it is likely that reactivated VZV passes to them. This hypothesized cause of post-herpetic pain may be in keeping with the Gate Control theory of pain of Melzack and Wall.

Viruses that may cause latent infections in humans are summarized in Table 5.2.

Latent virus infections including those due to HIV, EBV, and HSV have been among the latent virus infections that have been most firmly determined.

The mechanisms by which latent virus infections are established and the mechanisms of reactivation largely remain to be determined.

Table 5.2 Latent virus infections of humans

Virus	Primary illness	Cell type latently infected
Herpesviruses		
HSV-1,2	Cold sores genital infection	Sensory ganglion neurons
VZV	Chickenpox	Sensory ganglion neurons
EBV	Infectious mononucleosis	B lymphocytes
CMV	Infectious mononucleosis	Myeloid cells
HHV-6	Roseola	Probably monocytes
HHV-7	Roseola	Probably CD 4 lymphocytes
HHV-8	Fever, rash	Probably B lymphocytes
Retroviruses		
HIV	Varied	CD 4 lymphocytes
HTLV-1*	Varied	CD 4 lymphocytes

Table 5.2 (cont.)

Virus	Primary illness	Cell type latently infected
Polyomavirus		
JC virus	Often is asymptomatic	Kidney epithelial cells, brain cells
BK virus	Often is asymptomatic	Kidney epithelial cells
Papilloma virus	Asymptomatic, sometimes warts	Epithelial cells
Measles virus **	Measles	Neurons or other brain cells

* Human T cell lymphotropic virus type 1.

** It is not clear whether measles virus establishes a latent infection or a long-term, low-level persistent infection that leads to the illness subacute sclerosing panencephalitis (Chapter 7). Human adenovirus may cause a probably persistent infection in adenoid/tonsil cells that may periodically becomes more severe.

More is known of acute infections caused by these viruses. Acute, lytic infections are the focus of much research on antiviral medications and immunization. "Cure" of latent infections will likely require alternative medications and immune strategies.

Clinical aspects of viral pathogenesis and lytic infections of the nervous system are further discussed in Chapters 6 and 7. Chapter 8 returns to HSV latency and reactivation.

Further Reading

RT Gandhi, R Bedimo, JF Hoy, et al. Antiretroviral drugs for treatment and prevention of HIV infection in adults. *JAMA* 2023;**329**:63–84. https://doi.org/10.1001/jama.2022.22246

K Hoover, K Higginbotham. *Epstein Barr Virus*, StatPearls, 2021. www.ncbi.nlm.nih.gov/books/NBK559285/

AA Justiz Vaillant, PG Gluck. *HIV Disease Current Practice*, StatPearls, 2021. www.ncbi
.nlm.nih.gov/books/NBK534860/

A Richards, SH Berth, S Brady, G Morfini. Engagement of neurotropic viruses in fast
axonal transport mechanisms, potential role of host kinases and implications for
neuronal dysfunction. *Front Cell Neurosci* 2021;**15**:684762. https://doi.org/10.3389/
fncel.2021.684762

6

Viral Infections of the Nervous System

Various pathogens, including multicellular, unicellular, bacteria, viruses, and atypical agents, may cause illnesses of the human nervous system. Emphasis in this chapter is on viral infections of the nervous system.

Categories of Infectious Human Pathogens

Multicellular organisms
>   Helminths – tape worm
>   Fungi – histoplasma

Unicellular organisms
>   Protozoans – toxoplasma

Bacteria – streptococcus, pneumococcus, tetanus, Lyme disease

Viruses
>   DNA viruses – herpesviruses, smallpox virus, papilloma virus, polyoma virus
>   RNA viruses – retrovirus (for example HIV), corona virus (for example SARS-CoV-2), measles virus, influenza virus, mumps virus, poliomyelitis virus

Atypical agents

Viroids

Virusoids

Prions

Human Viruses

Virus classifications are often made on the bases of the viral genome, mode of replication, and viral morphology and not on the basis of illness caused, while clinicians and patients usually think in terms of organ systems.

For example, the family Picornaviridae (picornaviruses) includes poliomyelitis virus (there are three types of poliomyelitis virus) and coxsackie and echo viruses (8 types may infect humans). Polio viruses are classified as Group C Enteroviruses. Coxsackie and echo viruses are Group A and B Enteroviruses. These viruses cause gastrointestinal infections and may infect the nervous system.

Also included in the Picornaviridae family is the clinically very different rhinovirus group, the frequent cause of the common cold (there are more than 100 rhinoviruses reported to infect humans). To most clinicians and patients, a clinically related classification – which viruses may cause a polio-like syndrome versus which may cause an upper respiratory infection – is more important than a strict virological classification.

Similarly, in terms of clinical illness, five viruses have been reported to cause hepatitis. Of these, four are RNA viruses (or an RNA viroid) and one is a DNA virus, indicating they could not all be in the same family. They all may cause hepatitis, probably of more importance to patients and clinicians than their strict virology classification.

However, a virological classification may have clinical advantages in some situations. For example, including all herpesviruses as a group may not be intuitive when considering illnesses, but it may be helpful in some situations.

Herpes simplex virus (HSV) and Epstein–Barr virus (EBV) are both herpesviruses. As noted in Chapter 5, HSV causes latent infections of sensory ganglion neurons, and HSV may also cause encephalitis. EBV is considered to be in the category of infections of the lymphatic system. And as also noted in Chapter 5, EBV establishes latent infections of B lymphocytes. Although they cause different types of illnesses, considering these herpesviruses together may be useful when evaluating antiviral medications.

The following is a consideration of human viral infections with particular emphasis on infections of the nervous system.

Nervous system illnesses (viral or otherwise) are generally considered to be illnesses of the central nervous system (the brain and spinal cord) or of the peripheral nervous system (nerves, muscles), and there may be overlap between the two. Common clinical categories of infections of the nervous system include meningitis (infection, inflammation of the meninges, which cover the brain and spinal cord), and encephalitis (infection, inflammation of the brain).[54–57]

Individual viruses that infect the nervous system are discussed below, followed by discussion of viral meningitis and encephalitis.

Chapter 7 further discusses infections of the nervous system, including slow and latent virus infections. Also included are immunoinflammatory illnesses that may be triggered by viruses. Discussion there includes infection by atypical agents, particularly prions.

Viruses That Infect the Nervous System

Rabies virus – RNA virus. This virus is the cause of a well-described, very severe encephalitis with likely no survivors of this illness unless they are treated with the rabies vaccine (active immunization). Those exposed to rabies also often receive anti-rabies IgG (passive immunization). Rabies encephalitis is a lytic infection of brain cells. Emphasis has been on preventing rabies in animals, which decreases the spread to humans.

Veterinarians often receive rabies vaccine as a prophylactic preventive measure. Rabies virus is discussed in Chapter 5 as a virus that is transmitted from the periphery, for example, the site of an animal bite, to the brain by axoplasmic transport.[52]

Rabies was described in Mesopotamian literature, about 2000 BC.

ZOONOTIC VIRUS INFECTIONS

Rabies virus – Rabies is not a human virus in the sense of other viruses discussed here, such as HSV and EBV, which spread among people, but rather is an animal virus that occasionally infects and causes disease in humans and as such is zoonotic, meaning it may be transmitted from animals to humans. However, rabies is much more severe than most other zoonotic infections. Herpes B virus (discussed below) may also cause a severe zoonotic infection.

Influenza A is a zoonotic infection, transmissible from swine and birds to humans. Many arboviruses infections (discussed below) are indirectly zoonotic, being transmitted from infected animals to humans by insects such as mosquitos.

HUMAN VIRAL INFECTIONS

Poliomyelitis virus – RNA virus. This virus is the cause of clinical polio, usually meningitis accompanied by myelitis (inflammation of the spinal cord). The lytic infection may extend to include the lower part of the brain, the brainstem. Damage/destruction of motor neurons may occur in the spinal cord and the brainstem, and this may result in muscle weakness, including of muscles needed for breathing. The word "poliomyelitis" combines "polio" (from the Greek, meaning *gray* – the gray matter of the spinal cord, the neurons of the spinal cord) and "myelitis" (spinal cord inflammation). Poliomyelitis virus is one of the most important illnesses that have been controlled/eliminated by vaccines.

The very interesting and important post–polio syndrome[58] is further discussed in Chapters 7 and 9.

Poliomyelitis virus (types 1, 2, and 3) is a picornavirus, now classified as a Group C enterovirus. Coxsackie and echo viruses are Group A and B Enteroviruses. These enteroviruses often cause a primary gastrointestinal infection, hence the name "enterovirus." As is the case with many viral infections, infection may be asymptomatic or severe. Some individuals have no clinical history of clinical polio illness, but they have antibody to poliomyelitis virus in their serum. This suggests that they had had a subclinical or nonspecific gastrointestinal poliomyelitis virus infection. Before widespread vaccine use, the frequency of asymptomatic poliomyelitis virus infection, indicated by such seropositivity, was as high as 75% of the population.

Coxsackievirus and echovirus are probably the most common causes of viral meningitis. Uncommonly they cause myelitis or encephalitis. In recent years, there have been occasional reports of acute flaccid paralysis in children, and a possible connection to a Group D enterovirus, termed D68, has been investigated.

Enterovirus RNA was reported to be present by polymerase chain reaction (PCR) testing of spinal cord from amyotrophic lateral sclerosis (ALS) patients, but this has not been confirmed.

Herpes simplex virus – DNA virus. As discussed in Chapter 5, herpes simplex virus (HSV) frequently causes a latent infection of neurons of the trigeminal and dorsal root ganglia. With reactivation of HSV from latency, recurrent herpes labialis (face), keratitis (eye), and genitalis may occur. HSV type 1 (HSV-1) typically involves the face and HSV-2 the genital region. The former is due to latent infection and reactivation in trigeminal ganglion neurons, and the latter to similar infection and reactivation in sacral dorsal root ganglion neurons.

Cutaneous reactivated HSV infection can be treated and minimized with acyclovir (and related medications). However, latent HSV infection of neurons is not eliminated by acyclovir treatment.

HSV is also the cause of occasional encephalitis. HSV encephalitis typically involves the frontal and temporal lobes of the brain. In discussions below of encephalitis, a magnetic resonance imaging (MRI) of the brain of a patient with HSV encephalitis is presented (Fig. 6.1).

Varicella-zoster virus – DNA virus. Varicella-zoster virus (VZV) is in the herpesvirus family, and it is the cause of chickenpox in children and shingles (herpes zoster) in adults (Chapter 5). After initial chickenpox infection, latent infection may be established in sensory ganglion neurons (as for HSV). After viral reactivation, clinical shingles may occur. Shingles is more severe in older people, as is the pain of shingles. Pain after the occurrence of shingles may last for months/years and is termed "post-herpetic neuralgia." Vaccines are available to decrease chickenpox in children and to decrease shingles, and therefore prevent shingles pain in adults. Infection is somewhat treatable with acyclovir and similar medications.

Human herpesvirus 6, human herpesvirus 7 – DNA viruses. These herpesviruses (Chapter 5) are the cause of the childhood illness roseola (exanthem subitum). They are included here because, on occasion, they have been reported to be a cause of human encephalitis in people who are immunosuppressed. This point need be emphasized. When patients are immunosuppressed because of illness, for example, lymphoma, human immunodeficiency virus (HIV) infection, or because of medication they have received, viruses that ordinarily do not cause severe illness may cause severe illnesses such as encephalitis.

Similarly, adenovirus (DNA virus) encephalitis has occasionally been noted in immunosuppressed individuals.

Herpes B virus – DNA virus. This herpesvirus does not typically affect humans. It infects macaque monkeys and may be transmitted from them to humans, where it may cause severe encephalitis. It is the only nonhuman, primate herpesvirus that is pathogenic in humans. Herpes B encephalitis in humans emphasizes the caution that need be followed in handling animals, because of the possibility of infection of humans from animal viruses.

Herpes B virus infection of humans is a zoonotic infection that has the potential for causing severe illness.

Human immunodeficiency virus (HIV) – RNA retrovirus. HIV is the cause of illness of many organ systems, including the nervous system. Meningitis, peripheral neuropathy, spinal cord disease, and encephalitis are nervous system infections that may occur by HIV infection per se, and also by the many opportunistic illnesses that occur as a result of the HIV destruction of CD 4 T lymphocytes. Aspects of HIV pathogenesis are discussed in Chapter 5.

Human T cell lymphotropic virus type 1 (HTLV-1) – RNA virus. This human retrovirus is a cause of leukemia and lymphoma. In addition, after a period of viral latent infection (Chapter 5, Table 5.2), this virus may cause a severe demyelinating disease of the spinal cord, termed HAM (HTLV-1 associated myelopathy) or alternatively termed TSP (tropical spastic paraparesis). This spinal cord disease is noteworthy, in part, because the period of latent infection prior to spinal cord symptoms may be as long as 20 years.

Measles virus – RNA virus. The measles vaccine has been of great importance in decreasing the complications of measles virus infection. The past severity of measles complications in children should not be minimized. Acute measles (rubeola) encephalitis with severe sequelae was thought to occur in ~1/1,000. In addition, some children developed a slowly progressive encephalitis termed "subacute sclerosing panencephalitis" (SSPE) (Chapter 7).[59] Lastly, some developed a postinfectious encephalitis termed "acute disseminated encephalitis" (ADEM) (Chapter 7).

As noted in Chapter 1, it is thought that measles virus likely developed from cattle rinderpest virus, and that measles and canine distemper virus are closely related. Canine distemper virus is mentioned in discussing the epidemiology of multiple sclerosis in Chapter 7.

In the past, also before the advent of a vaccine, another childhood-acquired virus, mumps virus, was a common cause of viral meningitis.

Arboviruses – RNA viruses. This is a large group of viruses of different types that are transmitted by arthropods (**Ar**thropod **Bo**rne = Arbo), such as mosquitos, ticks, and sandflies (hematophagous, that is, blood-sucking insects). These viruses are often the cause of encephalitis and meningitis in the summer and early fall in North America and Europe.[10,56,60] Lyme disease is transmitted by ticks but is a bacterial rather than a viral infection.

Infections vary greatly, from asymptomatic to severe, the latter more so in the very young and the elderly. As is the case for many viral infections, infections by these viruses are often asymptomatic or mild. With some of these viruses, increased local animal infection, for example, horses infected with equine encephalitis virus, may be an indicator of increased risk of human infection.

Nonspecific initial signs of arbovirus infection often include fever, headache, fatigue, chills, and muscle pain. Nuchal rigidity (stiff neck), confusion, and focal neurological abnormalities may follow and suggest meningitis and encephalitis (discussed below). Treatment, as is often the case for viral infections, is symptomatic, that is, treating symptoms. With the development of antiviral medications and the availability of active immunization (vaccines) and possibly passive immunization (polyclonal and monoclonal antibody), specific treatments will become more available.

The following are all arboviruses, with this classification emphasizing their transmission from insects, even though the many viruses differ biochemically.

Several groups of arboviruses and some important viruses in these groups are outlined below:

Bunyavirus – California encephalitis virus, La Crosse encephalitis virus.

Togavirus – Eastern equine encephalitis virus, Western
equine encephalitis virus, Venezuelan encephalitis virus,
Chikungunya virus.

Flavivirus – Yellow fever virus, Dengue fever virus,[10] Japanese
encephalitis virus, St. Louis encephalitis virus, Tick-borne
encephalitis virus, Zika virus, West Nile virus.[56]

Zika virus is a flavivirus much discussed as a result of the 2015–2016
epidemic and the evidence that Zika virus was a cause of birth defects,
particularly microcephaly (small head–brain).[60]

Among the most important arboviruses through the world are yellow
fever virus and dengue fever virus, prevalent in tropical and subtropical
parts of the world.

While initial symptoms of yellow fever virus infection are often
nonspecific (as is the case with most arbovirus infections), illness may
proceed to more severe infection, resulting in jaundice – yellowing of the
skin due to elevated blood bilirubin, due to liver damage. Kidney damage
may also occur.

Vaccines are available to prevent infections by yellow fever virus,
Japanese encephalitis virus, dengue fever virus, and tick-borne
encephalitis virus. Vaccines are under development to prevent infections
by chikungunya virus, Zika virus, and West Nile virus.

It had been suggested by Carlos Finlay that yellow fever might be
transmitted by mosquitoes, and this was confirmed by Walter Reed.
Implementation of mosquito control to minimize yellow fever viral
infection was probably first instituted by William Gorgas in Havana and
in Panama. Evidence of mosquito transmission was a great advance in the
understanding of disease transmission and had a significant impact on
the development of the discipline of epidemiology.

The yellow fever virus was the first human virus to be isolated. A
vaccine to control yellow fever was developed by Max Theiler in 1937, and
for that he was awarded the Nobel Prize in Physiology/Medicine in 1951.

Viral Meningitis and Encephalitis

Meningitis may be caused by a number of viruses, bacteria and other pathogens. Meningitis is inflammation of the meninges, the coverings of the brain and spinal cord, with evidence of cerebrospinal fluid (CSF) infection. Meningitis symptoms include fever, stiff neck, photophobia, and headache. Intracranial pressure may be increased, with resultant confusion and possibly coma. CSF will be abnormal, and increased intracranial pressure can be determined by measuring CSF pressure. CSF is discussed in Chapter 7.

Encephalitis is less common than is meningitis and is inflammation of the brain – sometimes there may also be myelitis (inflammation of the spinal cord). Encephalitis symptoms usually include the symptoms of meningitis plus confusion, coma, seizure, and focal neurological symptoms, such as hemiplegia. With damage to the brain and spinal cord, many types of neurological symptoms may occur. CSF is abnormal, similar to meningitis. Given some of the overlap between meningitis and encephalitis, it is common for patients to be diagnosed with meningoencephalitis.

Viral meningitis is more common than is viral encephalitis.[54,55,57] Viral meningitis has often been referred to as aseptic meningitis, because using usual methods of CSF culture, virus that might be present was not detected. Historically, the usual culture methods were designed to permit the growth (the isolation and detection) of bacteria. Unless living cells are used, viruses will not be isolated. PCR testing of CSF has greatly enhanced the ability to identify specific viruses and other organisms that cause meningitis and encephalitis.

The viruses most often responsible for viral meningitis are the nonpolio picornaviruses, such as the coxsackieviruses and echoviruses. These viruses uncommonly cause encephalitis. The arboviruses occasionally cause viral meningitis but are of greater concern in instances of viral encephalitis. Infections by enteroviruses and arboviruses typically occur during the summer and early fall months in temperate climates.

PARANEOPLASTIC (AUTOIMMUNE) ENCEPHALITIS

Patients with cancers of varied types may develop inflammatory illness of the nervous system termed "paraneoplastic encephalitis." Sometimes the encephalitis is focal or somewhat focal such as limbic encephalitis (hippocampus, hypothalamus, amygdala), cerebellitis (cerebellum) and brainstem. Importantly, some patients will present with the encephalitis before they are diagnosed with the cancer. Oftentimes antibodies thought to be cross-reactive between the tumor and the nervous system are found, including anti-GAD, anti-Hu, and anti-NMDA receptor antibodies. Immunosuppressive treatments are minimally or not at all helpful, although improvement is often seen with treatment of the cancer. Autoimmune encephalitis is further discussed in Chapter 7.

Case Report

Confusion may be the presenting symptom of viral encephalitis, as exemplified by the following case.

The author was asked to review the medical history of a patient diagnosed with HSV encephalitis. The patient was a 23-year-old male who was confused and brought to a local hospital emergency department for evaluation. The following is from the medical record:

There was no pertinent past medical history and no history of recent injury or illness.

Respirations were 22 and regular. Pulse was 92 and regular, and blood pressure was 118/67.

The patient was slightly drowsy but followed most commands. He was not oriented to place but was to year. His speech was rambling and dysarthric.

He was normocephalic without evidence of injury. His neck was supple. Eye movements were full and pupils symmetrical and reactive. There was no facial asymmetry. There was no arm or leg weakness or sensory loss. DTRs [deep tendon reflexes] were slightly increased but were symmetrical and there were no pathological reflexes.

Screening tests including blood count, liver function, kidney function, glucose, and urinalysis were normal. Chest x-ray and computerized tomographic (CT) scan of the brain were normal.

Further testing of the patient's urine came back positive for marijuana.

The patient was discharged with the diagnosis of confusion related to marijuana toxicity.

He was no better the next day and so was brought to a different emergency department. There was no significant change in the history or physical examination. A brain MRI was performed and was abnormal and consistent with HSV encephalitis.

The patient's family brought a legal case against the first hospital, charging them with medical malpractice.

HERPES SIMPLEX VIRUS (HSV) ENCEPHALITIS

HSV, usually HSV-1, is a nonseasonal cause of viral encephalitis. The temporal and frontal lobe predilection for HSV encephalitis has been noted in many instances (Fig. 6.1). To explain this finding, some have suggested reactivation of HSV in trigeminal ganglion neurons and transport from that site to the frontal and temporal lobes, although there is no clear anatomical pathway. From evidence of experimental HSV latent infection of the brain (Chapter 5), it is suggested that human HSV encephalitis may result from reactivation of occasional HSV latent brain infection.

Unlike the treatments of other viral causes of encephalitis, which are largely supportive, acyclovir is very useful for the treatment of HSV

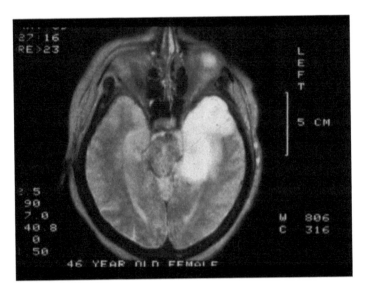

Figure 6.1 Brain MRI (magnetic resonance imaging) in a patient with HSV encephalitis, with particular left temporal lobe damage (heavy white signal). In MRI images, the viewer's right is the left side of the brain of the patient.

encephalitis. For that reason, many patients who present with apparent encephalitis start receiving acyclovir, which is often continued for several days. It is very safe, and it (and similar medications of its class) are often used to initially treat encephalitis patients, even when the specific cause of encephalitis is not found; there is little downside to it use.

HIV may cause a viral meningitis, usually early in the course of the illness, and encephalopathy, as part of AIDS, may occur later after HIV infection in those who are untreated. The frequency of AIDS has greatly decreased with effective HIV antiviral medication use.

Lymphocytic choriomeningitis virus (LCM), a rodent virus, is an occasional cause of human meningitis. As noted above, the consideration of types of organisms that may cause meningitis and encephalitis need be greatly expanded in evaluating immunosuppressed individuals.

Birth Defects

Birth defects as a group is not an organ system per se, although the brain is often involved. It is included here as a separate entity because of its importance. Among the viruses that are important in considering birth defects are human cytomegalovirus (a herpesvirus), rubella virus, herpes simplex virus, and Zika virus.[60,61] LCM, discussed above as a possible cause of meningitis, may also cause birth defects.

Cytomegalovirus (CMV) – DNA virus. Subclinical CMV infection is a particular issue during pregnancy, because many mothers may not be aware of their having a CMV infection during pregnancy. Infection of the fetus may cause microcephaly, inflammation of the retina, hearing loss, and seizures. Non-neurological abnormality may include liver damage with accompanying jaundice. CMV is also a known cause of a mononucleosis-like syndrome in children and young adults.

Rubella virus – RNA virus. Rubella virus–related birth defects are somewhat of a lesser concern than in the past, because of the wide availability and use of the rubella virus vaccine. Prior to the vaccine availability, abnormalities of vision, hearing, and heart were noted. Rubella virus infection was of particular concern when the infection occurred during the first trimester of pregnancy. Testing of women for antibody to the virus before pregnancy is advised, with women receiving the vaccine if they do not have rubella antibodies. Live virus vaccines such as the rubella vaccine are usually not administered to pregnant women (Chapter 4).

Herpes simplex virus (HSV) – DNA virus. This virus (usually HSV-2) is particularly an issue when infants are born through an HSV-infected birth canal. HSV-2 reactivation from lumbosacral dorsal root ganglion neurons is likely the cause of recurrent genital HSV infection. While such HSV infection may be clinically apparent, sometimes it is not.

Zika virus – RNA virus. This virus in the large arbovirus group has been noted in recent years as a cause of birth defects, particularly microcephaly in newborn infants.[60]

Atypical Illnesses and Agents

ENDOGENOUS RETROVIRUSES

A type of "unusual infection" of the nervous system and other organ systems relates to the presence of endogenous retroviral elements. In summary, humans (and other animals) have in the DNA of their cells genes that were apparently derived from retroviruses, probably millions of years ago. Possibly 5% of human DNA is thought to be derived from these viruses. Human retroviruses, in the form of DNA proviruses, are integrated into human DNA (Chapter 5). Such retroviruses are RNA viruses, and so our DNA contains DNA provirus copies of these viruses.[62]

These retroviruses have been termed "endosymbionts" by some investigators. In some instances, the endosymbiotic benefit to the pair of organisms (the host and the endosymbiont) seems apparent. As noted in Chapter 3, the mitochondria of cells have been considered as endosymbionts – where there is benefit to the endosymbiont organism and to the cells in which they "infect."

We can speculate on possible advantages to human (and other animal) cells that led to these retrovirus sequences being incorporated into human DNA. It is easier to see the advantage from the retrovirus viewpoint, in that the sequences (at least parts of the retrovirus) are increased by the trillions of copies in human and animal cells.

Endogenous retroviral elements in humans may be thought of as remote (in terms of human evolution) infections, whereby viral RNA genetic information became incorporated in the form of a DNA provirus into our genome. The concept of endogenous retroviruses blurs the concept of infection.

It has been investigated whether these retroviral elements may play a role in human cancer and in human illnesses (for example, amyotrophic lateral sclerosis, multiple sclerosis).

Endosymbionts may be an example of the concept of "selfish DNA." The concept of selfish DNA was introduced by George Williams and Richard Dawkins, in considering that some genes seem to reproduce themselves preferentially. One might think generally of nucleic acids that can reproduce themselves, such as RNA and DNA (Chapter 3), as being inherently selfish.

VIRUSOIDS

Virusoids (satellite virus, defective virus) contain RNA and protein, but the gene for the virusoid protein is not encoded in its RNA. It is encoded and supplied to the virusoid by a helper virus. The agent that causes hepatitis D has been considered a virusoid. Hepatitis D infection only occurs in people also infected with the hepatitis B virus, and the hepatitis D agent uses some hepatitis B virus functions to replicate. The occurrence of hepatitis D infection only with concomitant hepatitis B infection raises the possibility of similar coinfections, by other virusoid–virus combinations.

VIROIDS

Viroids (satellite nucleic acids) are infectious naked RNA particles, without protein. These simple pieces of naked RNA replicate using cellular biochemical machinery. Although these subviral, very simple infectious agents replicate, they further push the concept of "aliveness."

It would be a real stretch to conclude that they are living forms. They are included here as being virus-like agents.

PRIONS

If we can argue whether viruses, virusoids, and viroids are alive, the prion argument is whether disease caused by these "replicating things" can be considered infections (probably not). It is not possible to consider them as being alive. Prions are an exception to the concept of "infection" by organisms that replicate via Central Dogma methods (Chapter 3). These "infectious" proteins contain neither RNA nor DNA.[21] Prion diseases are discussed in Chapter 7.

SLOW AND LATENT VIRUS INFECTIONS

Not so bizarre as viroids, prions and endogenous retroviruses are the concepts of slow and latent viral infections. Slow infections would be expected to demonstrate at least low levels of virus replication, while latent virus infections would be expected not to demonstrate virus replication (Chapter 5).

If during slow virus infections, low levels of virus replication are present, low-level persistent infections and slow virus infections might be thought similar. A slow virus infection of the nervous system, subacute sclerosing panencephalitis (SSPE) due to measles virus,[59] is discussed in Chapter 7.

Latent virus infections caused by HIV, EBV, and HSV are discussed in Chapter 5, and experimental HSV latency is further discussed in Chapter 8.

As noted in Chapter 5, concluding that an infection is a latent infection rather than a slow infection (a qualitative difference) may depend on a quantitative difference (how much viral protein or viral reproduction can be detected). If viral protein and viral reproduction are not detected, which would suggest a latent infection, is it only because sensitive enough methods were not used?

Important in any discussion of latent virus infections where viral reactivation may occur are considerations of stimuli that may cause reactivation.

Speculation on the Reactivation of Latent Virus Infections

As discussed in Chapter 5, the occurrence of HSV latent infection in the trigeminal system was first suggested by the neurosurgery procedures of Harvey Cushing. He noted clinically apparent HSV reactivation (facial HSV infection) after trigeminal root (Fig. 5.1) surgery for the treatment of trigeminal neuralgia. This was probably the first clear evidence of a cause of viral reactivation.

In subsequent years, rather than cutting the trigeminal root, other neurosurgical procedures were developed to treat trigeminal neuralgia. These included trigeminal root/ganglion decompression, but also compression (with glycerol or mechanically). It seemed that multiple methods to "stimulate" the trigeminal ganglion were effective. Equally interesting is that all the procedures resulted in the occurrence of HSV reactivation. It has been suggested that physical stimulation of latently infected trigeminal ganglion neurons resulted in HSV reactivation.

One of the most interesting and well-documented causes of HSV reactivation is ultraviolet (UV) light, which seems to cause reactivation that is site specific. That is, reactivation occurred at sites that received the UV light.

Reactivation of HSV-1 and HSV-2 has been suggested to occur at times of stress, to be related to hormone changes, and to occur after immunosuppression. Reactivation of VZV and the occurrence of herpes zoster (shingles) has been similarly related to these. One can speculate as to whether these stimuli cause viral reactivation or whether they cause replication of reactivated virus.

That is, do those stimuli result in reactivation at the level of the latently infected neuron, or do they result in enhanced replication of virus that had reactivated for other reasons? The author believes that evidence of HSV after trigeminal system neurosurgery is due to reactivation at the level of the latently infected neuron. But it is likely that evidence of HSV (and probably VZV) infection after stress, immunosuppression, and hormonal change is the result of enhanced replication of virus that has reactivated for other reasons.

Clinically asymptomatic reactivation of HSV, with shedding of infectious virus, has been well described. Stimuli that cause such reactivation are not known. It is suggested that if such "spontaneous" viral reactivation were to occur at times of immunosuppression, stress, or hormonal change, enhanced virus replication would occur, and it would seem that those stimuli caused the reactivation. These conclusions remain to be investigated.

A second interesting issue of uncertainty relates to viral reactivation in latently infected neurons. It might be thought that with reactivation and the synthesis of virus in neurons, those neurons would be destroyed. Production of infectious virus within a cell generally produces cell lysis. While severe zoster (shingles) may result in cutaneous sensory loss (indicating neuron loss – Chapter 5), that is not usually the case for mild zoster and for HSV reactivation.

With reactivation of HSV and VZV, it is thought that virus nucleocapsids (virus particles without the viral envelope) or fully enveloped virus particles travel via axoplasmic transport (Chapter 5) from the neuronal cell body to skin/mucous membrane surfaces. Asymptomatic shedding of infectious virus or localized skin/mucous membrane infections results. Although fully infectious virus is present, neuron loss, suggested by areas of sensory loss, is not typical.

Further Reading

WT Jackson, CB Coyne. *Enteroviruses: Omics, Molecular Biology and Control*, Caister Academic Press, 2018. Book 978–1–91090–73–9, Ebook 978–1–91090–74–6

S Said, M Kang. *Viral Encephalitis*, StatPearls, 2021. www.ncbi.nlm.nih.gov/books/NBK470162/

Q Wang, YJ Tao. *Influenza: Current Research*, Caister Academic Press, 2016. Book 978–1–91090–43–2, Ebook 978–1–91090–44–9

7

Neurovirology and Immunology

This chapter continues discussion of viral infections of the nervous system and includes discussion of neuroimmunology, including neurological illnesses that may triggered by viruses.

Neurovirology

While viral infections of the nervous system such as rabies (including the development of the rabies vaccine) were known in the nineteenth century, and arbovirus infections were described in the early twentieth century, many consider the start of neurovirology to be in the 1950s. It is not so much viral infections of the nervous system that define neurovirology, but rather the concepts of slow and latent virus infections, as well as atypical infections of the nervous system.

Second, investigations and insights of the possible role of viruses in triggering autoimmune illnesses of the nervous system were actively being developed in the 1950s, and 1960s. Therefore, neurovirology and neuroimmunology have often been considered together.

Paradoxically, prions that do not contain RNA or DNA are usually included under the heading of neurovirology. It is startling that illnesses caused by prions, which do not contain nucleic acid, not only may be genetically transmitted within families, but also can "infect," that is, can be transmitted to experimental animals.

Many studies in the area of neurovirology have related to investigations of a possible viral cause of multiple sclerosis (MS), which is an autoimmune illness. Virus investigations in MS continue, particularly the possible role of Epstein–Barr virus (Chapter 5), human herpesvirus 6, and endogenous retroviruses. MS investigations have often emphasized the epidemiology of this illness, which has seemed consistent with an infectious cause – in the United States and in Europe MS is more frequent in northern latitudes.

While MS is an autoimmune demyelinating disease of the central nervous system (CNS) – the brain and spinal cord – Guillain-Barré syndrome is an autoimmune demyelinating disease of the peripheral nervous system (PNS) – the peripheral nerves. Myelin, made by different cell types in the CNS and in the PNS (Chapter 5), serves as an electrical insulating material in both, and myelin facilitates electrical transmission in the nervous system.

Human Illness after Viral Infection and after Immunization

Case Report

Some years ago, the author was asked by a U.S. attorney to evaluate the medical record of a 62-year-old woman (Mrs. XX) who developed leg weakness ~5 weeks after having received influenza virus immunization.

The following is from her medical record:

The patient described leg weakness, initially involving her right foot. Over 3 days, it progressed to involve both feet and both legs. She noted difficulty voiding but no difficulty with bowel movements. There was numbness of her feet. She denied weakness or numbness of her hands–arms and had no facial weakness or numbness. She denied loss of vision, double vision, difficulty with chewing, swallowing, or speaking.

There was no history of headache or other pain. There was no history of recent illness or injury.

There was no history of prior neurological symptoms.

Her health was generally good. She had hypertension that was controlled with diuretic medication.

On physical examination, vital signs (pulse, blood pressure and respirations) were normal. There was no evidence of injury, and she had no pain. She was alert and cooperative. The general physical examination was benign.

The neurological examination showed intact speech. Vision, eye movements, and pupil responses to light were normal. Hearing was intact. There was no facial or arm weakness or numbness. The patient could not stand without assistance. Both legs were weak and there was numbness to just above the knees. Deep tendon reflexes (DTRs) were normal in her arms and increased in both legs [discussed below].

The patient was diagnosed as having Guillain-Barré syndrome, due to the influenza immunization she had received.

Review of the Case

There was a disconnect between the diagnosis of Guillain-Barré syndrome and her increased leg DTRs. In brief, DTRs would be expected to be decreased and certainly not increased with Guillain-Barré syndrome, an illness of the PNS.

For that reason, she was examined, about 6 months after the onset of weakness. The results of the neurological examination were similar to the medical record information.

The patient's leg weakness had improved, and she was able to walk with a walker. The DTRs in her arms were normal and they were still brisk in both legs. A positive Babinski reflex (upgoing great toe with plantar stimulation) in the right foot and a probable positive Babinski reflex on the left were present.

It was concluded that her leg weakness may well have been due to the influenza immunization, but she did not have Guillain-Barré syndrome (a PNS illness). She likely had developed myelitis (sometimes termed "transverse myelitis"), spinal cord inflammation (a CNS illness), which caused her leg weakness.

This case might be a good example of the issues of data and the interpretation of data.

Influenza Immunization and Guillain-Barré Syndrome

Subsequent to large numbers of people receiving influenza virus immunization in the 1970s and in later years, it was noted that there was some relationship between having received the vaccine and the development of Guillain-Barré syndrome.[63]

The incidence of Guillain-Barré syndrome in the general population (without prior influenza virus immunization) was thought to be about 2 per 100,000 population. With the influenza immunization, the incidence was about 4 per 100,000. Therefore, the incidence doubled, but it was still only ~4 in 100,000 people. Given the low incidences involved, to detect an effect of the influenza immunization may be thought of as an epidemiological triumph.

In a recent interesting study of patients who had a history of prior Guillain-Barré syndrome and were immunized with an mRNA vaccine to prevent COVID-19, 1 out of 702 developed a mild relapse.[64]

Post-Infectious Neurological Illness

Over many years it has been concluded that some patients who develop Guillain-Barré syndrome have had an antecedent clinical event or illness. The antecedent event may have been an injury or surgery or an illness. In some, the event appeared to have been immunization. In many patients, no clear antecedent event was apparent, and in some of these it was often thought that the individual may have had a mild asymptomatic viral illness.

Illness such as Guillain-Barré syndrome occurring after a viral infection is often stated to be a post-infectious illness (sometimes termed "para-infectious"). The implication is that the antecedent illness altered the patient's immune system, and that the immune system then "attacked" the patient's nervous system. Autoimmune illness resulted, such as Guillain-Barré syndrome (PNS illness) or myelitis (CNS illness).

Interesting in considerations of the pathogenesis of Guillain-Barré syndrome, possibly due to such immune overreactivity, are the occasional reports of Guillain-Barré syndrome occurring in immunosuppressed individuals, for example, kidney transplant patients. In these instances, an autoimmune illness occurred during a time of immunosuppression.

In addition to influenza virus as an antecedent event to Guillain-Barré syndrome, antecedent human cytomegalovirus (CMV) and Epstein–Barr virus (EBV) are often considered as triggers of the autoimmune illness. Both are herpesviruses that establish latent infections and that may reactivate (Chapter 5). Also associated with the development of Guillain-Barré syndrome are antecedent infections by *Campylobacter jejuni*, *Mycoplasma pneumoniae*, and *Haemophilus influenzae* (all are bacteria).

A common hypothesis to explain immunologically mediated neurological illnesses after infection or after receiving a vaccine is that of molecular mimicry. It suggests that some of the many amino acid sequences of proteins in the infecting organism or in the administered vaccine may be similar to amino acid sequences of cellular proteins, for example, in myelin. Therefore, when the host immune system recognizes these sequences in the infecting organism or vaccine, and B and T lymphocytes are activated, the immune system ends up attacking myelin in the vaccine recipient. The mimicry might occur at the 3-dimensional level where even if specific amino acids are not the same, the 3-dimensional structure might be similar. Molecular mimicry is a compelling explanation for post-infectious or vaccine-induced autoimmunity.

Molecular mimicry probably had its origin from observations that cardiac valve disease followed rheumatic fever caused by streptococcus bacteria. Heart valve damage was thought to be due to immunological cross reactivity between bacterial antigens and cardiac valve tissue.

In addition to the occurrence of peripheral nerve (PNS) illness such as Guillain-Barré syndrome after viral infection or immunization, CNS inflammatory illness may occur. Myelitis and brain inflammation may occur. The latter is sometimes termed "acute disseminated encephalomyelitis" (ADEM).

ADEM is more frequent in children than in adults and is typically a monophasic event, and multiple sclerosis is more frequent in adults and is typically multiphasic. Discussion of multiple sclerosis (CNS illness) after illness and immunization follows.

Mrs. XX may well have developed leg weakness due to the influenza immunization she received, but she did not develop Guillain-Barré syndrome. This is confidently stated due to her brisk leg DTRs. In Guillain-Barré syndrome, the DTRs are decreased or absent, while they are increased (brisk) after myelitis. Guillain-Barré syndrome and myelitis both may result in leg weakness, but the former is an illness of the PNS and myelitis is an illness of the CNS.

A brief discussion of the nervous system, particularly the CNS (involved in MS) and the PNS (involved in Guillain-Barré syndrome) follows.

The Nervous System

The nervous system consists of the CNS (brain, spinal cord) and the PNS (nerves, muscles). The brain consists of a very large number of neurons (nerve cells), which communicate with one another by way of long axon, cellular extensions (Chapter 5). Communication from neuron to neuron is electrical, and electrical activity can be recorded from the brain in the form of an electroencephalogram (EEG). Nerves that project to the muscle cells of the heart regulate the heart rate and rhythm, which along with the electrical activity of the heart muscle cells can be recorded in the electrocardiogram (EKG).

Chemicals act as intermediaries between the axons of neurons and the cell membranes of other neurons. Electrical activity in axons causes the release of the chemicals (neurotransmitters). Upon release from axon terminals, these neurotransmitters bind to receptors in the neurons being contacted, which causes new electrical activity in those neurons.

Alternatively, neurotransmitter released from the axons of motor neurons (neurons which project to muscle cells) binds to receptors of muscle cells. This alters electrical activity in the muscle cells, which results in the muscle cells contracting.

The axon terminal and the membrane of the neuron or muscle cell being contacted by the axon form a synapse. The axon terminal is said to be presynaptic, and the neuron or muscle membrane receiving the neurotransmitter is postsynaptic.

At the peripheral ends of motor axons, the chemical acetylcholine is released, which crosses from the axon terminal to the muscle cell – a synapse termed the "neuromuscular junction." Acetylcholine uptake by receptors in the muscle cell membrane results in electrical changes in the muscle cells, and the muscle cells contract, resulting in movement.

As discussed in Chapter 5, the symptoms of botulism result from botulinum toxin inhibiting the release of acetylcholine from axon terminals. Therefore, electrical activity is not generated in the muscle cells, and they do not contract.

Since the nervous system is largely an electrical system, there should be no surprise that insulation is present. The insulating material is myelin made by oligodendrocytes in the CNS and by Schwann cells in the PNS. Importantly, the myelin that oligodendrocytes make is chemically different from that which Schwann cells make.

Damage to myelin (demyelination) in the CNS or PNS results in altered or blocked transmission of electrical impulses and the occurrence of altered neurological function.

Guillain-Barré syndrome, a PNS illness, is due to damage to Schwann cell myelin. Multiple sclerosis (MS) a CNS illness, is due to damage to oligodendrocyte myelin. Both MS and Guillain-Barré syndrome are often thought of as inflammatory autoimmune demyelinating illnesses that may be triggered by viral infections. Myelitis, as in the case of Mrs. XX, may occur as part of MS or as a single episode of CNS demyelination.

Inflammatory Illnesses of the Nervous System

Inflammatory illnesses of the nervous system may be due to infectious or noninfectious causes. As was discussed for viral infections (Chapter 6), infections may cause meningitis, encephalitis, and myelitis. And as part of these syndromes, inflammation of nerves (nerve roots) leaving the brain and spinal cord may also occur. All of these types of inflammatory conditions may also occur due to noninfectious causes such as autoimmune illnesses.

Noninfectious, autoimmune causes of brain, spinal cord, and meningeal inflammation include illnesses such as MS, sarcoidosis, systemic lupus erythematosus, and a group of illnesses termed "paraneoplastic illnesses." Guillain-Barré syndrome is a noninfectious, autoimmune illness of nerve roots.

Before considering specific illnesses, one last background section, on cerebrospinal fluid (CSF), is presented. In patients with MS, Guillain-Barré syndrome, myelitis, meningitis, and encephalitis, CSF testing is often performed. It also may be tested in patients with Alzheimer's disease and many other inflammatory/degenerative illnesses of the nervous system. The CSF may reveal much about the nervous system.

Cerebrospinal Fluid (CSF)

Cerebrospinal **fluid (CSF)** is made in the four ventricles of the brain – the two lateral ventricles (right and left), and the two midline, third and fourth ventricles. CSF flows from the ventricles to bathe the brain and the spinal cord, and it is absorbed into the bloodstream at the top of the brain. The CSF provides nutrients to the brain and physically cushions and supports it. Humans have 125–150 ml of CSF and make ~300–400 ml per day, so it is continuously being replenished. When the flow of CSF is obstructed, the pressure in the ventricles increases, the ventricles enlarge, and hydrocephalus ("water on the brain") results.

In considering inflammatory and infectious illnesses of the nervous system, sampling of the CSF often provides important clinical information. CSF is obtained by lumbar puncture (spinal tap). The first measurement performed is the CSF pressure. Normal pressure is less than 200 mm of CSF. Subsequent CSF studies typically performed include total protein, immunoglobulin G (IgG), red blood cells, white blood cells (WBCs), and culture for bacteria. Polymerase chain reaction (PCR) testing may be performed on CSF to determine the presence of viruses, bacteria, and other infectious agents.

With bacterial infections of the nervous system, bacterial meningitis, there is an increase in the number of WBCs in the CSF – sometimes a very great increase. And the increase is usually due primarily to increase in the number of polymorphonuclear WBCs. With viral meningitis, the increase in WBCs is usually less dramatic, and the increase is likely to be due primarily to an increase in lymphocytes.

The CSF glucose may be decreased and the CSF total protein increased with infections. The decreased glucose and the increased total protein abnormalities are more likely to be present and more likely to be severe with bacterial than with viral infections.

With bacterial infections, the offending organism may be isolated in culture, while this is not usually true for viral infections, the reason for the historical conclusion that viral meningitis was "aseptic" – as discussed in Chapter 6. PCR testing has become very important in permitting the identification of specific infectious agents causing meningitis and encephalitis.

Other studies are often performed on CSF, depending on clinical circumstances, for example, cytology if a neoplasm is suspected. Emphasis in the present discussion is on studies of CSF IgG.[65]

In evaluating patients for inflammatory or possible autoimmune illness of the nervous system, the amount of IgG in CSF is often measured. This is usually the chemical measurement of the amount of IgG present. It is not the biological measurement of IgG antibody directed against a particular antigen, such as neutralizing antibody.

However, biological measurement of CSF IgG antibody to a particular antigen such as a virus protein antigen can be performed. In such instances, the question is often whether the CSF IgG antibody against the viral antigen was made in the CSF, or whether it was made in the blood and "leaked over" into the CSF (discussed below).

In MS patients, CSF IgG is increased (chemical measurement), and it has been found to be directed against many antigens (biological measurements), suggesting general B lymphocyte activation, rather than B lymphocyte activation against a particular antigen. CSF IgG measurements in MS are usually of the total amount of IgG (chemical measurement) and not measurements of IgG against specific protein antigens (biological measurements).

THE BLOOD–BRAIN BARRIER (BBB)

Although the blood that nourishes all organs and the CSF are in equilibrium, they are in separate fluid compartments. Virtually all chemicals found in the blood are also present in the CSF. With few exceptions, the amounts in the CSF are less than in the blood. However, with brain/spinal cord inflammation–infection–injury, the equilibrium is altered and the BBB is breached. This may occur with encephalitis, meningitis, tumor, stroke, or head injury. Breaching (breaking) the BBB results in increased CSF amounts of probably all chemicals that are present in the blood – although CSF amounts are still less than in the blood.

A common clinical question is whether the increase in a substance in the CSF (for example, IgG) is due to increased amounts of it being made in the CSF, or due to breach of the BBB.

THE IGG INDEX

For both MS, where the amount of chemical IgG is measured, and for viral infections where the amount of IgG biologically active against the virus may be measured, whether the IgG was made in the periphery and "leaked over" into the CSF or was made in the CSF compartment can be determined.

For example, consider a viral infection. If the infection is outside the CNS, such as in the lungs, IgG against the virus (biological measurement) will be present in the blood, and a small amount would be expected to leak over into the CSF. If the infection is within the CNS, such as viral encephalitis, a greater amount (biological measurement) of IgG against the particular virus will likely be present in the CSF.

Whether IgG against a particular virus was made in the blood (as the result of a lung infection) and spilled over in small amounts into the CSF or was made in the CSF can be investigated, based on several measurements. The investigation can be initiated based on the observation that the normal ratio of IgG in blood (serum) to CSF IgG is about 140:1.

This ratio is based on the following:

Total protein in serum is about 7 grams per deciliter (dL), that is 7,000 mg per 100 ml.

Total normal CSF protein is about 50 mg per 100 ml.

7,000/50 = 140:1, a useful starting approximation, which can be refined with real measurements.

Therefore, if a patient had been infected, for example, with West Nile encephalitis virus but did not have clinical meningitis/encephalitis (intact BBB), it would be expected that the patient would have IgG antibody to the virus in the blood (biologically measurement), and about 1/140 of that amount in the CSF. Antibody to the virus would be made in lymph nodes and in the blood, and a small amount of that antibody would have spilled over into the CSF.

However, if the patient had West Nile meningitis or encephalitis, since IgG against the virus (biological measurement) would also be made in the CSF compartment, the amount of antibody against the virus in CSF would be greater, and the ratio of biologically measured IgG in serum to CSF would be decreased. The absolute amount of serum IgG antibody against the virus (biologically measurement) would likely still be greater in the blood than that in the CSF antibody against the virus, but the ratio would be decreased.

More accurate calculations can be made by measuring the serum total protein rather than estimating it to be ~7,000 mg per 100 ml, and also measuring the CSF total protein rather than assuming it to be ~50 mg per 100 ml.

The same considerations occur in evaluating the chemical measurement of CSF IgG of patients with MS, much more common than the biological measurement of CSF IgG against a virus. The following is the usual means to measure the amount of chemical IgG in CSF in MS patients, and to determine whether any increase is due to a leaky BBB or due to IgG being made in the CSF – the determination of what is termed the IgG Index.

Rather than simply measuring the total amount of CSF IgG, which had been done in the past, accuracy is enhanced with two corrections. Since CSF IgG might be increased because the amount of IgG in the blood is increased (for example, myeloma), likely resulting in the leak of greater amounts of IgG into the CSF, a serum IgG correction is needed. Since CSF IgG might be spuriously increased because the BBB is not intact, resulting in the leak of all proteins in the blood into the CSF, including IgG, a CSF protein correction is needed.

The CSF IgG Index calculation in multiple sclerosis (chemical measure of IgG) is the ratio of the CSF IgG to the serum IgG divided by the ratio of the CSF total protein (or albumin) to the serum total protein (or albumin) (or total protein) (Table 7.1).[62]

Table 7.1 CSF IgG Index calculation in multiple sclerosis

CSF IgG/serum IgG	(corrects for possible increased IgG in serum [uncommon])
―――――――――――――――	
CSF total protein/serum total protein	(corrects for possible leaky BBB [common])

CSF IgG measurement of this type is routinely performed in considering autoimmune illnesses of the nervous system such as MS. The formula in Table 7.1 is used to determine whether CSF IgG is increased, and if so whether it was due to the IgG being made in the CSF.

Rather than measuring the amount of chemical IgG (for MS studies), biological measures such as neutralizing antibody titer of IgG against specific antigen (such as the West Nile virus) could be performed with similar corrections to determine whether specific IgG against the virus was made in the CSF or leaked over from the serum.

Several specific viral illnesses of the nervous system are considered in the following, prior to a return to discussions of MS.

Neurological Viral Illnesses

Discussion of latent virus infections as compared with lytic infections was introduced in Chapter 5. As noted there, with lytic infections, virus replication and viral products (proteins) are evident – although this might be slight with some low-level persistent infections. With latent infections, virus replication is not evident.

SLOW VIRUS INFECTION: SUBACUTE SCLEROSING PANENCEPHALITIS (SSPE)

The illness subacute sclerosing panencephalitis (SSPE) has been termed a slow virus infection, due to a type of measles virus infection.[59] The illness typically occurs after measles infection of young children, and the illness is unusual in that it often does not present until years, sometimes 10 or more, have passed. Speculation has centered on the role of a possible abnormal immune response in young children as well as on abnormal measles virus. The panencephalitis of SSPE includes both demyelination and neuron loss.

The concept of slow virus infections raises consideration of an unusual type of infection with unusual pathogenesis. It is thought that in SSPE the measles virus infection is persistent (rather than latent) and becomes clinically manifest years later.

A striking characteristic of SSPE is the large amount of IgG antibody to measles virus (biological measure) that is present in the CSF of patients. The ratio of anti-measles antibody in CSF to serum (see above discussion of CSF IgG Index) is probably the largest of any known clinical illness.

SSPE was an uncommon type of measles infection that has become more uncommon after the advent of the measles virus vaccine.

Less common than the uncommon illness SSPE is progressive rubella panencephalitis. This illness resembles SSPE but is caused by rubella virus, usually after congenital rubella or childhood rubella infection.

It had been known for years that with a chronic infection of the nervous system, for example, syphilis (neurosyphilis), antibody to the infecting agent was greatly increased in the CSF. SSPE is a viral infection of the nervous system where this is evident. Since increased CSF IgG is a characteristic of MS, the increased CSF IgG in SSPE supported considerations of MS being due to a virus infection. However, in SSPE the increased CSF IgG is directed against the measles virus, and in MS the increase is not against any single antigen.

LATENT VIRUS INFECTIONS

These are viral infections that are maintained in cells without evidence of viral replication. On occasion, however, the latent virus may reactivate with subsequent evidence of viral replication. The neurosurgical stimulus for the reactivation of HSV from human trigeminal ganglion neurons is discussed in Chapter 6. For the most part causes of viral reactivation are not known; as discussed in Chapter 6, it is unclear if stimuli such as immune suppression cause viral reactivation or permit the replication of virus that was reactivated for other reasons.

Latent viral infections have been best described for the human herpesviruses and for human retroviruses, including HIV, and possibly less clearly so for human polyoma and papilloma viruses.

Herpes Simplex Virus, Varicella-Zoster Virus, Epstein–Barr Virus, and HIV

Latent infections caused by these viruses are discussed in Chapters 5, 6, and 8. The latent infections established by these viruses are probably the best defined among the examples of human virus latent infections. During latency, the DNA genomes of the three herpesviruses exist as intranuclear episomes,[46] and the RNA genome of HIV exists as an integrated DNA provirus.

Human Polyoma Viruses: BK and JC Viruses

BK virus and JC virus were so named from the initials of the people from whom they were first isolated.

BK VIRUS INFECTION

BK virus does not usually cause infection of the nervous system, and it is discussed here because it probably causes latent infections and because of its similarities to JC virus (which does cause neurological illness – discussed below). BK virus infects most people (as indicated by elevated serum antibody to the virus in most people), and it establishes a latent infection in the kidney. Approximately 90% of people are seropositive for BK virus, suggesting they had been infected with that virus at some time.

BK virus may reactivate with pregnancy, as evidenced by increased serum antibody (IgM and IgG). It is likely the latent virus infection reactivates and the repeat infection results in increased IgM and IgG. As noted in Chapter 4, antibody increase after infection is first of the IgM antibody class, and after a period of time IgG antibody increases.

Increase in antibody titer of, for example, from 1:64 (usually stated as 64) to 1:1,024 (1,024) suggests reinfection or is due to the reactivation of a previously latent viral infection. A 4-fold (or greater) increase in the antibody titer is usually considered clinically significant and evidence of repeat infection.

Evidence of BK virus reactivation during pregnancy is sometimes also directly evidenced by the shedding of virus in the urine of pregnant women. BK virus has been shown to reactivate particularly in immunosuppressed people, including after kidney transplant, sometimes leading to failure of the transplant.

JC VIRUS INFECTION: SLOW VS LATENT VIRUS INFECTION

JC virus is similar to BK virus and is also common in the population. About 75% of people are seropositive for the virus. The virus is latent, with specifics as to cell type(s) latently infected and the nature of the viral genome during latency yet to be clearly determined. Most studies have suggested the kidney and lymphocytes as sites of latency.

In addition to kidney latency, there is also evidence that JC virus may be latent in brain cells, including of normal people. It is possible that subsequent to immunosuppression, viral reactivation from those cells leads to the demyelinating illness of the brain, progressive multifocal leukoencephalopathy (PML).

There is also evidence that as part of the reactivation process of JC virus from latency, more neurotropic virus variants may be selected, and this neurotropic virus results in infection of oligodendrocytes and demyelination.[67,68] The concept of viral variants being selected in specific tissues during infection of those tissues had been discussed in the 1980s.[7]

As noted in Chapter 5, JC virus causes the CNS demyelinating illness PML. The occurrence of this illness is related to immunosuppression. PML was greatly increased by the AIDS pandemic.[66-68] In PML, oligodendrocytes are infected by the JC virus, and the destruction of these CNS myelin-producing cells results in demyelination.

Significantly, some patients with MS have developed PML, likely the result of immunosuppressive medication they received to treat their MS. These individuals have CNS demyelination due to their MS and CNS demyelination due to PML.

Although JC virus infection is being described as a latent rather than a slow or persistent virus infection, one can see the general issue. As discussed, a slow (or persistent) infection would be accompanied by evidence of virus replication, and a latent infection would not. But the evidence may depend on the detection methods used and their sensitivity.

Striking areas of demyelination occur in PML. While immunosuppression is often a precipitating factor leading to PML, and MS patients are not immunosuppressed, the concept of a virus that causes a demyelinating disease of the human CNS had been important in considering MS, a demyelinating illness of the CNS.

Figures 7.1 and 7.2 show postmortem results of brain tissue testing from an immunosuppressed patient (due to lymphoma) diagnosed with PML. Figure 7.1 shows many JC virus particles in the brain, as seen by electron microscopy. Figure 7.2 shows blot DNA testing of brain tissue, confirming that the virus seen was JC virus.

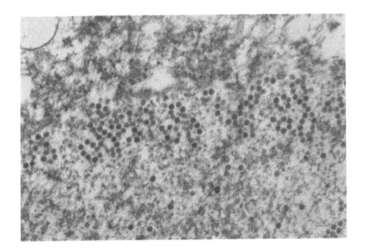

Figure 7.1 Multiple JC virus particles, 41–43 nm in diameter (electron microscopy magnification 75,000) in brain tissue obtained at postmortem from a patient with PML. From Tenser RB, et al. *J Neurol Sci* 1986;**72**:243–254. Used with permission, Elsevier.

JC virus is very difficult to grow in cell culture, usually requiring culture with a type of fetal cell. For that reason, other methods have been developed to identify the virus, for example, using DNA methods. For the conclusion that the virus seen in Figure 7.1 was JC virus, viral DNA from brain tissue was cut with several restriction endonucleases, as was the prototype known JC virus, and the resulting DNA fragments were compared. They are the same size (Figure 7.2).

Multiple Sclerosis (MS)

From the last quarter of the twentieth century, there have been many studies in attempts to find a possible viral cause of MS, a demyelinating disease of the CNS, in which CNS myelin (made by oligodendrocytes) is

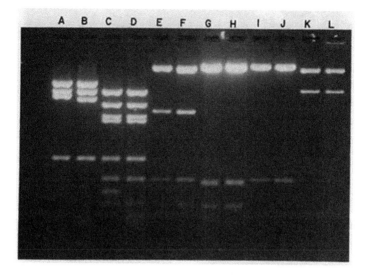

Figure 7.2 Electrophoresis pattern of pairs of DNA fragments, after restriction endonuclease cleavage of prototype Mad 1, JC virus DNA (left in each pair), and postmortem brain PML viral DNA. The similarity of the DNA restriction fragments from the prototype JC virus and from the postmortem virus confirms the presence of JC virus in the brain tissue. From Tenser RB, et al. *J Neurol Sci* 1986;**72**:243–254. Used with permission, Elsevier.

destroyed. The demyelination results in impaired transmission of signals from neurons to neurons. The areas of demyelination are very varied throughout the CNS, resulting in very varied symptoms.

Frequent, however, are demyelination of the optic nerves, resulting in impaired vision, demyelination of cerebellar and brainstem pathways, resulting in impaired limb and eye coordination, and demyelination in the spinal cord, resulting in leg weakness, sensory loss, and impaired bladder control. (Although termed a nerve, the optic nerve is part of the brain, the CNS, and it is not part of the PNS.)

Among the reasons why MS was thought to possibly have a vial etiology were immunological, virological, and epidemiological observations.

The first clearly defined laboratory test abnormality in MS was the presence of increased IgG in CSF. Not only is the IgG total increased, but it usually is in the pattern of oligoclonal bands. These are multiple, discrete concentrations of IgG made by what are often termed B lymphocyte clones. One might think of MS oligoclonal IgG as several monoclonal antibodies made by groups of B lymphocytes.

As noted above, the detection of increased CSF IgG and oligoclonal bands were noted with neurosyphilis. Therefore, the observation of oligoclonal bands in MS suggested a possible infectious cause. More to the point is the very elevated CSF IgG in SSPE, a chronic measles infection of the brain, as described above.

In addition, canine distemper virus, a virus related to measles virus, causes demyelinating brain lesions in dogs, and so there were further considerations of a possible viral cause of MS.

These virological observations, coupled with the epidemiological observations of increased MS in northern latitudes throughout the world, supported investigations of a possible viral cause of MS.

EPIDEMIOLOGY OF MS

It has been known for a number of years that MS affects some populations more than others. For example, it affects women more than men.

In the United States, the prevalence of MS is estimated to be about 1/1,000 population. There is some genetic basis of MS, and if one person in a family has MS, siblings of that person have about a 3–4% chance of having MS. That is increased to ~30–35% in identical twins.

Multiple sclerosis is more frequent in northern latitudes (in the northern hemisphere). What about people who move? There is some evidence that for people moving from a northern high incidence area to a southern low incidence area, or vice versa, age may be important. Moving before about age 15 seemed important. If moving after that age from a high incidence area to a low incidence area, individuals retained the high incidence. Similarly, if moving from a low incidence area to a high incidence area after about that age, individuals retained the low incidence.[69]

The northern latitude increased incidence was consistent with a possible infection, and the age-related moving data suggested important early life events – and maybe a slow-moving virus infection.

Several viruses, including human herpesvirus 6 and particularly Epstein–Barr virus (EBV), have been potentially linked to MS.[70] A part of the virus-related hypothesis is the concept of early life infection versus later life infection. Some have thought that in western cultures people are too clean, which diminishes early life exposure to infections. This might be bad if later exposure produces a severe or an abnormal response. This is the hygiene hypothesis.

For example, EBV infection in infants may be benign, but later infection may result in clinical infectious mononucleosis. There is consideration that later life initial EBV exposure may result in an abnormal immunological response, with clinical MS as the result.

Considering a possible role for EBV in the pathogenesis of MS has also been attractive for the reason that EBV infects B lymphocytes,[51] important in MS.

After exposure to an antigen, B lymphocytes synthesize IgG antibody to the antigen (Chapter 4), and excessive IgG (made by B lymphocytes) is present in the cerebrospinal fluid (CSF) in patients with MS (see Table 7.1 and text discussion). B lymphocytes are also important in that they present antigen to T lymphocytes, the cell type that causes demyelination in MS.

As introduced in Chapter 5, EBV vaccines are in early stages of development. In terms of MS, it will be necessary to consider whether an EBV vaccine should be given to children to try to prevent an illness hypothesized as being related to EBV, and which occurs in ~1 per 1,000 people. As is the case with all medications/vaccines, consideration of the risk:benefit ratio is important.

In part related to measles virus in SSPE studies and the demyelination produced by the measles-like canine distemper virus, epidemiological studies were performed on MS patient dog ownership. Initial studies showed no clear relationship. What about dog size? It was thought that on average, large dogs were more likely to live outside in dog houses and small dogs more likely to live in the house. Small dogs, therefore, might be the link with MS. However, controlling for dog size did not show a relationship.

Lastly was the dog urine hypothesis, which was to take into account a possible role of distemper or similar virus and the northern latitude affect. It considered that there might be a virus (distemper or similar) that infected dogs. When dogs urinated on the sidewalk, people would be potentially exposed to the virus. In the north, the rays of the sun were less direct, and therefore when dogs urinated on the sidewalk, the virus was less likely to be inactivated than in the south, where the rays of the sun were more direct.

Current emphasis on the effect of latitude on MS is related to sunlight and vitamin D – greater in southern than in northern latitudes.

The cause of MS continues to be unknown. Emphasis is that it is an autoimmune illness, with recent focus moving away somewhat from a T lymphocyte emphasis and to a greater B lymphocyte emphasis.

MS EXACERBATION VS PSEUDO-EXACERBATION

Clinical exacerbations (relapses) of MS are related to new demyelinating events. New symptoms occur or prior symptoms are worsened. Similarly, new brain/spinal cord abnormalities may be seen on MRI scans. These clinical and MRI abnormalities are thought to be the result of a new autoimmune demyelinating events. For the most part, causes of exacerbations are not known. Some have suggested they may follow illnesses, possibly subsequent to illness-related immune system activation. MS exacerbations may follow the inhibition of the cytokine tumor necrosis factor, which inhibition is useful to treat rheumatoid arthritis, another autoimmune illness. And interferon gamma was noted to worsen MS.

Pseudo-exacerbations are clinical occurrences of the worsening of preexisting MS symptoms, and they are most commonly noted when MS patients have illnesses with fever. Decrease of the fever results in the rapid improvement of pseudo-exacerbation symptoms. Similar pseudo-exacerbations may also occur at the time of other illnesses. Pseudo-exacerbations are likely the result of MS-damaged CNS structures being physiologically impaired by fever/illness, with rapid improvement following correction of the abnormal physiology.

CAN VACCINES CAUSE MS?

With epidemiological evidence that vaccines may be associated with autoimmune illness such as Guillain-Barré syndrome, there has been consideration of a possible association of vaccines with MS.[71]

Several years ago, the author was asked by an attorney at the U.S. Department of Justice to review the case of a young woman who received the papilloma virus vaccine to prevent cervical carcinoma, and who said that she then developed MS.

The occurrence of illness such as MS after vaccine immunization have generally emphasized two possibilities.

One suggested possibility is the occurrence of immunologically mediated damage to nervous system tissue (myelin) resulting from molecular mimicry. As discussed above, the molecular mimicry hypothesis suggests that some protein antigens in a vaccine and in myelin are similar, and that the host immune response to antigens in the vaccine damages host cells and tissues.

Another suggestion relates to vaccines enhancing nonspecific immune reactivity. For example, the release of cytokines may occur in vaccine recipients, and this has been hypothesized as leading to autoimmune illness. It is of interest that blocking tumor necrosis factor (a cytokine that is abnormally elevated in the autoimmune illness rheumatoid arthritis) may worsen MS. And although MS may improve after beta interferon treatment, it may worsen after treatment with interferon gamma.

NATIONAL VACCINE COMPENSATION PROGRAM

In the 1980s, the U.S. government established the National Vaccine Injury Compensation Program (NVICP). It had been recognized that vaccines are important for individuals and for the population, and enhanced vaccine use would be a positive for the populace. Vaccine use would be a win-win, in that it would improve health and would decrease medical expenses.

It was recognized, however, that some individuals are reluctant to use vaccines because of "side effects" – some real and some not so much. It was also thought that vaccines were not a priority of pharmaceutical companies, in part because they were a target for legal actions when side effects were noted. The NVICP would shift liability from pharmaceutical companies to the government.

The NVICP is a no-fault program whereby 1. listed vaccines that are covered are noted, 2. listed complications that are covered are noted, and 3. the time interval between vaccine receipt and complication occurrence is indicated. If the three criteria are appropriately met, coverage is provided.

For example, if after seasonal influenza virus immunization an individual develops Guillain-Barré syndrome, and the onset is between

3 and 42 days after receiving the vaccine, compensation is provided. Legal cases may arise when any of the three criteria are not clearly met.

Information about the vaccine program can be accessed at www.hrsa .gov/vaccine-compensation/index.html.

The case the author reviewed was of a patient who had brought a legal challenge. The general medical issues with cases such as hers were whether the patient had the illness being cited (that is, was the MS diagnosis accurate) and whether the time interval between the vaccine immunization and the development of the illness was reasonable.

The accuracy of diagnosis issue returns to Mrs. XX discussed in the Case Study, who upon review was thought to not have Guillain-Barré syndrome but rather myelitis. But the illness of Mrs. XX did occur shortly after the vaccine was received, and her development of myelitis was probably related to the influenza immunization.

In the present papilloma virus vaccine case, when the medical records of the woman were examined, there was clear evidence of MS. The diagnosis was well supported by abnormal clinical examination findings and abnormal laboratory test findings. However, she had received the papilloma vaccine 15 months previously. Cases of MS after papilloma virus vaccine had been reported in Australia, with an average interval of 21 days between vaccine receipt and illness onset.

As noted above, the prevalence of MS in the general population is about 1 in a 1,000. Was the patient in question in the 1/1,000 group or was the MS occurrence due to the vaccine?

A second issue that might be considered in MS cases is whether a vaccine "caused" MS or rather caused an exacerbation of preexisting, possibly subclinical MS. This would lead to consideration of whether factors that cause the onset of MS are similar to factors that cause exacerbations (relapses) of MS. This issue came up in cases where MS occurred (or subclinical MS was exacerbated) when patients were treated with tumor necrosis factor (TNF) inhibitors.

THE TREATMENT OF MS

The treatment of MS has advanced greatly and will not be discussed at any length here. Most treatments have emphasized immunosuppression, becoming more sophisticated with time to have a T lymphocyte or a B lymphocyte focus. Treatment has been of great clinical value, although "cure" remains elusive.

However, some patients do seem to be "cured" – in that they do not report new clinical episodes and their brain MRI is unchanged. Of course, in some patients these findings occur without treatment. Unclear is the time duration necessary prior to claiming a cure has occurred. Again, the issue is the data (no clinical worsening, no MRI worsening) and the interpretation of the data.

It is apparent that early treatment of MS is important. And in this regard, MRI developments have been invaluable. While in the past, the diagnosis of MS was clinically based and often required years of follow-up, in recent years, MRI abnormalities have sometimes sufficed to permit the diagnosis after an initial single clinical episode. Early diagnosis has become frequent, and this has had a very important effect on describing the MS clinical course, including the efficacy of medication.

Earlier diagnosis of an illness such as MS sometimes requires new consideration of the natural history of the illness. In some ways this may be the application of the Will Rogers Phenomenon to medicine.

The Will Rogers Phenomenon as Applied to Medicine: Data and the Interpretation of Data

Will Rogers was an American humorist. In the 1930s, he made a statement having nothing to do with medicine or science, which was cleverly applied to medicine by Alvan Feinstein.

Will Rogers, in commenting on people from the American Dust Bowl, such as those from Oklahoma (the Oakies) who in the 1930s moved to California to seek better lives, said, "When the Oakies left Oklahoma and moved to California, they raised the average intelligence level in both states."

Alvan Feinstein was an epidemiologist. Among his studies were investigations of survival times of groups of cancer patients, including cancer patients with metastases (cancer that had spread to other sites) and those without metastases. It comes as no surprise that the average survival in the latter group was greater than in the former.

He then noted the use of a new diagnostic technique to investigate possible metastases, positron emission tomography (PET). This technique detected even very small metastases.

Some patients thought not to have metastases by conventional testing methods did in fact have metastases – that could only be seen by PET scan. He placed these patients, who previously were in the nonmetastatic disease group, in the metastatic disease group.

The remaining nonmetastatic disease group now only had definitive nonmetastatic disease patients. Therefore, the average life expectancy of the nonmetastases group was increased.

Patients with the very small PET-determined metastases were placed in the metastases group. But the metastases they had were very small – only detected by PET scan. For that reason, the average survival of patients in the metastases group was longer than prior to adding those patients to the group.

The average life expectancy of people in both groups was increased – described by Feinstein as the Will Rogers Phenomenon.

This can be seen in the following very hypothetical example.

If the average life expectancy is:

5 years for people with no metastatic disease

4 years for people with only PET evidence of metastatic disease – they have very small metastases

3 years for people with other more overt evidence of metastatic disease

Consider 7 patients, 3 with no metastatic disease (each indicated with a 5), 3 with clear evidence of metastatic disease (each indicated with a 3) and one with only PET evidence of metastatic disease (indicated with a 4).

The use of PET testing would result in moving the single "4" patient from the no metastases group to the metastasis group. As seen in Table 7.2, without PET evaluation, the single "4" patient would be in the No metastatic disease group and with PET evaluation would be in the Metastatic disease group.

Moving the patient from the nonmetastatic disease group to the metastatic disease group because of PET evidence of metastatic disease increased the average life expectancy of both groups – the Will Rogers Phenomenon.

The issue of such improved diagnostic methodology on predicting the clinical course of an illness can be applied to much of medicine. In the diagnosis of MS, MRI testing has led to earlier diagnosis. This may result in MS patients seeming to do better over time from disease onset than in the past. Methodology that results in earlier diagnosis of an illness may seem to improve the patient course after diagnosis. This application of the Will Rogers phenomenon has been noted for MS.[72]

As emphasized in several places in this volume, there are data and then there is the interpretation of the data.

Table 7.2 Life expectancy of nonmetastatic and metastatic disease patients

Without PET evaluation		With PET evaluation	
Nonmetastatic disease group	Metastatic disease group	Nonmetastatic disease group	Metastatic disease group
5, 5, 5, **4**	3, 3, 3	5, 5, 5	3, 3, 3, **4**
Ave. life expect. 4.75 years	Ave. life expect. 3 years	Ave. life expect. 5 years	Ave. life expect. 3.25 years

Post-Polio Syndrome

It was noted that some patients who had polio years in the past developed increased weakness. Some patients who had residual weakness from polio 30–40 years previously developed new weakness. It seemed like worsening polio.[58]

An initial consideration of course was that the poliomyelitis virus had been latent for those many years, and then had reactivated and was causing reinfection and damage of motor neurons.

This concept was also important for investigations of amyotrophic lateral sclerosis (ALS), a severe neurological illness with some features that resemble clinical polio. In both illnesses, large spinal cord motor neurons (neurons that project from the spinal cord to muscles) are specifically damaged/destroyed, although in ALS additional structures are also involved.

Several studies did not show evidence of residual or latent poliomyelitis virus. Virus reactivation or a slow virus infection was not thought to be the cause of the post-polio syndrome.

It was concluded that post-polio syndrome was due to an interesting and in some ways novel pathological mechanism. It is thought that clinical polio years previously had "subclinically" damaged spinal cord motor neurons. And now years later, that mild neuron damage, possibly plus the usual changes of aging, manifested as motor neuron death. Motor neurons had been damaged years previously, and now those neurons were dying. Increased muscle weakness was the result.

Unlike other cell types in the body, most neurons do not divide, and this is clearly the case for motor neurons. Therefore, the motor neurons that you were born with are the neurons you now have. The idea of prior damage from an agent (for example, polio) and then the superimposition of the ravages of time is an intriguing concept.

Prion Illnesses: Kuru, Creutzfeldt–Jakob Disease, and Other Spongiform Encephalopathies

Vincent Zigas was a physician who in the 1950s evaluated an unusual illness in the Fore people of the Papua New Guinea highlands. People had developed an apparent neurodegenerative disorder, with a greater incidence in children and women. There appeared to be a relationship of the disorder to ritualistic cannibalism, and cannibalism caught the eye of the public.

As part of a ritual honoring the deceased individual, cannibalism was practiced. Women and children more often ate the brain tissue of the deceased than did men. Some developed an illness, usually with a latency of years. Symptoms included shaking, poor coordination, and mental deterioration. The illness was named Kuru, which meant "shaking" in the language of the Fore.

Zigas was joined by Carleton Gajdusek, and they published an extensive study in 1957 on what they termed a degenerative disease of the central nervous system. However, the illness seemed transmissible – very unusual in concept for a degenerative illness – and was thought to result from the ritualistic cannibalism practiced. There was much discussion of whether it was transmitted by the cannibalism per se, or possibly by handling the brain tissue and having the transmission occur through open sores or wounds on the face or hands.

EXPERIMENTAL TRANSMISSIBILITY OF KURU, CREUTZFELDT–JAKOB DISEASE, AND SCRAPIE

Over subsequent years, Gajdusek showed that the illness could be experimentally transmitted. He did this by inoculating brain material from patients with Kuru into the brains of experimental animals. This demonstrated the "infectivity" and transmissibility of a degenerative condition. Gajdusek received the Nobel Prize in Physiology/Medicine in 1976 for this work.

The brain pathology of Kuru was like that of a presumed human degenerative illness, Creutzfeldt–Jakob disease. Patients with Creutzfeldt–Jakob disease presented with personality change, dementia, hallucinations, and incoordination. After studies of the experimental transmissibility of Kuru, human Creutzfeldt–Jakob disease was also shown to be transmissible to experimental animals.

It was thought that Kuru likely started with a Fore individual developing Creutzfeldt–Jakob disease. Then it spread as the illness Kuru from that individual to others through the ritualistic cannibalism practice. With the discontinuation of cannibalism, Kuru disappeared.

In other studies, it was noted that the brain pathologies of Kuru and Creutzfeldt–Jakob disease were similar to that of the animal disease scrapie. All had areas of loss of brain substance with a spongy appearance of the brain, and they were all classified as spongiform encephalopathies.

Scrapie is a disease of sheep and goats and had been known since the mid-eighteenth century. A disease of deer and elk, chronic wasting disease, is similar.

In subsequent years, many experimental studies were performed with scrapie brain material. Extensive studies showed that scrapie could be transmitted to mice using brain material from scrapie-diseased animals. Significantly, the brain tissue that was shown to transmit scrapie did not appear to contain DNA or RNA. Eventually, it was concluded that transmission of scrapie was by a protein.

Very significantly, it was possible to breed knock-out mice that do not have the specific normal cellular protein. If these animals, lacking the normal protein, were inoculated with scrapie material, they did not develop scrapie. Therefore, even when inoculated with the abnormal scrapie protein, the absence of the specific normal protein prevented the development of scrapie.

PRIONS

From multiple studies, it was concluded that scrapie and the related spongiform illnesses are caused by a specific, abnormally configured protein. And this abnormally configured protein causes normal protein to become abnormally configured. This returns to the concept of the importance of the 3-dimensionsal configuration of proteins (Chapter 3).

In the knock-out mouse studies, it was demonstrated that if the specific normal protein is not present, the abnormal scrapie-causing, abnormally-configured protein will not cause scrapie – there is no protein substrate for the abnormal scrapie protein to alter. There is no increase or "replication" of abnormal protein. Stanley Prusiner won the Nobel Prize in Physiology/Medicine in 1997 for his work in this area.

The abnormal protein has been termed a prion. The scrapie prion behaves like an infectious agent in that is seems to multiply. Hypothetically, for example, if 100 units of the scrapie agent (the abnormal protein) are inoculated into an animal, over time the animal will develop scrapie. And since the abnormal scrapie protein has caused a specific normal protein to become abnormal, there is an increase in the amount of abnormal scrapie protein. There are now 1,000 units of the abnormal scrapie protein. It has increased in amount, similar to the increase of infectious organisms after infection.

Most cases of human Creutzfeldt–Jakob disease are sporadic, but 5–10% are familial, with the illness being transmitted as an autosomal dominant abnormality. Human spongiform illnesses similar to Creutzfeldt–Jakob disease include Gerstmann–Sträussler–Scheinker disease and fatal familial insomnia. These illnesses are due to genetic abnormalities, and as is the case with familial Creutzfeldt–Jakob disease, they may be transmitted within families. Such genetic transmission is not a surprise since many illnesses may be genetically transmitted.

Abnormal genes result in abnormal proteins, and abnormal genes may be transmitted in families. What is amazing, however, is that these genetic illnesses can be transmitted to experimental animals, like infections, similar to scrapie.

MAD COW DISEASE

In the 1980s, bovine spongiform encephalopathy, colloquially known as mad cow disease, was described in the United Kingdom. An illness of cattle was thought to have occurred following the feeding of cattle with scrapie-containing bone meal from scrapie-infected sheep, and in effect caused scrapie in cattle. The peak incidence was in 1993. Spread to humans by the eating of meat from these cattle caused what was termed variant Creutzfeldt–Jakob disease. It is thought that ~290 people developed this illness.

Variant Creutzfeldt–Jakob disease caused impaired coordination, dementia, and psychiatric symptoms, with an average life span of ~1 year. It was similar to usual Creutzfeldt–Jakob disease, although it occurred in people younger than those who usually developed that illness. As might be expected, this occurrence caused great upset, and animal care was subsequently greatly altered throughout the world.

Chronic wasting disease of deer (also elk, moose) appears to be another prion disease of the nervous system. The author is not aware of disease transmission to humans following the consumption of meat from these animals.

IATROGENIC TRANSMISSION OF CREUTZFELDT–JAKOB DISEASE

In addition to the transmission of Creutzfeldt–Jakob disease to humans as part of the mad cow episode, transmission has occurred several times through medical care. For example, transmission occurred after dural patch surgery, where dura was used to cover the site of brain surgery. The dura is a covering over the brain. Sometimes dura is harvested after death of an individual and used in the surgery of another individual.

Similarly, transmission of Creutzfeldt–Jakob disease occurred after corneal transplant surgery, using the cornea from a deceased individual. Transmission also occurred following growth hormone replacement, where growth hormone was prepared from deceased individuals.

Lastly, transmission of Creutzfeldt–Jakob disease was thought to have occurred after use of intracerebral electrodes to record the electrical activity of the brain. Even though the electrodes used had been sterilized after use in a previous patient, transmission seemed to have occurred.

In these instances, it is thought that the deceased individuals from whom the dura, cornea, and growth hormone were obtained had unknown Creutzfeldt–Jakob disease. Use of such human donor biological materials has undergone much scrutiny, and controls are much improved since these occurrences.

The electrode-mediated transmission of Creutzfeldt–Jakob disease emphasizes unique properties of prions as compared to viruses, bacteria, and other infectious organisms – the electrodes had been sterilized by usual surgical methods. However, prions are resistant to conventional sterilization procedures, although they are sensitive to chemicals such as bleach. It is now general practice to discard surgical instruments used in the evaluation/treatment of patients with possible with Creutzfeldt–Jakob disease, rather than attempting sterilization and subsequent use in another patient.

CREUTZFELDT–JAKOB CASE REPORT

The Neurology consultation team was asked to evaluate a 74-year-old woman on the Psychiatry service.

The patient had abnormal behavior for 1 to 2 months. Her speech was halting with occasional inappropriate words. There was no recent injury or illness. The was no history of loss of consciousness or seizure.

On exam, the woman showed no evidence of injury, and the general physical examination was benign.

The patient spoke haltingly but without dysarthria. She responded to questions with speech but did not initiate speech. She followed some simple commands – close your eyes – but not those minimally more complex – raise your right arm. She could not subtract 7 from 10.

Eye movements were probably benign, and pupils were minimally but symmetrically reactive. There was no facial asymmetry. There was no weakness of her arms or legs and sensation was grossly intact. DTRs were probably normal. However, with each DTR test, the patient had a total body jerk. She had similar body jerks (termed "myoclonus") in response to a loud sound (for example, the examiner clapping hands). There was no evidence of abnormal plantar reflexes, but the patient was not cooperative.

Brain MRI showed slight atrophy. Electroencephalogram (EEG) testing showed slowing with high-voltage waves, particularly on the left. Periodic high-amplitude waves were present with myoclonus. She was thought to have Creutzfeldt–Jakob disease.

Elevated levels of a protein termed 14-3-3 protein have been found in the CSF of some patients with Creutzfeldt–Jakob disease. However, this abnormal protein has not been found to be specific for Creutzfeldt–Jakob disease. More promising is the euphonious, Real-time Quaking-Induced Conversion Test. This test uses test cerebrospinal fluid from a patient and known normal protein. If abnormal prion protein is present in the cerebrospinal fluid, it serves as a nidus, and normal protein is converted to abnormal. Abnormal protein accumulates, and it is easily detected.[73]

Figure 7.3 shows a brain section of a patient with Creutzfeldt–Jakob disease.

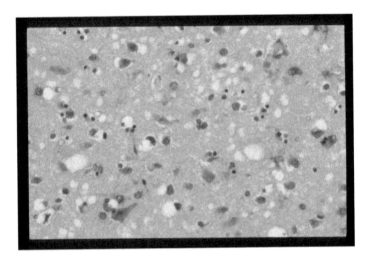

Figure 7.3 Spongiform encephalopathy in Creutzfeldt–Jakob disease. Multiple vacuolated abnormalities within and around brain cells are seen, giving the brain the characteristic "spongy" appearance.

NONTRANSMISSIBLE PRION DISEASES?

Kuru and Creutzfeldt–Jakob disease were initially thought to be human degenerative diseases. With time, they were found to be caused by transmissible prions. Some might consider them as infectious diseases, but if so, they are clearly different from all others. They may be considered as infectious-degenerative illnesses – a new category of illness.

More recently, other degenerative illnesses have been evaluated for the possibility of having a similar pathogenesis. Some have thought of illnesses such as Alzheimer's disease and Parkinson's disease as being caused by prion-like proteins. Abnormal proteins are known to accumulate in these illnesses, but transmissibility has not been demonstrated.

Therefore, it has been considered that these and possibly other illnesses may be due to prion-like proteins, but to be different in that they are not transmissible. They might be due to abnormal proteins that accumulate by causing normal proteins to become abnormal, but to not be transmissible.

The concepts of protein causing other protein to become abnormal and the possible of "infectivity" of proteins alter concepts of both infectious and metabolic/degenerative illnesses.

Further Reading

H Lassmann, Pathogenic mechanisms associated with different clinical courses of multiple sclerosis. *Front Immunol* 2019;**9**:3116. https://doi.org/10.3389/fimmu.2018.03116

E Leitzen, BB Raddatz, W Jin, et al. Virus-triggered spinal cord demyelination is followed by a peripheral neuropathy resembling features of Guillain-Barré syndrome. *Sci Rep* 2019;**9**(1):4588. https://doi.org/10.1038/s41598-019-40964-1

A Sakudo, T Onodera, eds. *Prions: Current Progress in Advanced Research*, Caister Academic Press, 2019. Book 978–1-91090–95-1, Ebook 978-1-910190–96-8

8

Experimental Neurovirology

This chapter on experimental herpes simplex virus (HSV) infection of the nervous system builds on information presented in Chapter 5 on viral pathogenesis. Emphasis here is on HSV latent infection of neurons and neuronal factors important for viral reactivation from latency.

HSV Latent Infection

As introduced in Chapter 5, latent viral infections are not simply low-level infections by viruses such as HSV, varicella-zoster virus (VZV), Epstein–Barr virus (EBV), and human immunodeficiency virus (HIV) but rather are different types of infections. During latency, viral genomic nucleic acid is in an altered state, and infectious virus is not produced. As discussed in Chapter 5, while the entire HSV DNA genome is present during latency, only a single viral RNA, the latency associated transcript (LAT) is expressed.[46] Questions relate to the mechanisms by which latent infections are established and the events and mechanisms by which reactivation from latency occurs.

Acyclovir

In 1988, Gertrude Elion won the Nobel Prize in Physiology/Medicine, in part for her work on the mechanism of action of the antiviral medication, acyclovir. Acyclovir is very useful in the treatment of HSV and VZV infections and was probably the first true antiviral – a medication that was specific for these viruses.

As noted in Chapter 3, acyclovir is a nucleoside analog, and as is the case with such medications, it is a pro-drug that needs to be biochemically altered to function as an antiviral.[29] The alteration necessary is that it be phosphorylated – a phosphate group (PO_4) need be added. This is performed by the enzyme thymidine kinase (TK).

Animal cells, including human cells, contain two TK genes and, therefore, two TK enzymes – a cytosolic TK (TK1) and a mitochondrial TK (TK2). TK was introduced in Chapter 3 in considering mitochondrial myopathy. Cellular TK1 is present in small amounts in most neurons (nondividing cells) and in increased amounts in dividing cells such as cancer cells.[74,75]

HSV also has a gene for its own TK – it codes for a viral TK. Importantly, acyclovir is "recognized" by the HSV TK but not by the cellular TKs – mitochondrial or cytosolic. As part of this recognition process, HSV TK phosphorylates the pro-drug acyclovir, and in the phosphorylated form, acyclovir impairs HSV DNA replication. Phosphorylated acyclovir is incorporated into growing HSV DNA, instead of thymidine deoxynucleotide. This damages the growing viral DNA, and virus replication is blocked.

Acyclovir greatly inhibits the growth of HSV and limits HSV lytic infections. However, HSV latent infections are not eliminated by acyclovir, presumably because during latency the virus is not replicating.

Cell TK is limited in what it will phosphorylate (only thymidine deoxynucleoside and uridine ribonucleoside), while HSV TK is said to be promiscuous, in that it will phosphorylate many substances, including acyclovir.

As is the case for acyclovir, remdesivir, and molnupiravir (which have been tested for antiviral use in the treatment of SARS-CoV-2 infections) are pro-drug nucleoside analogs and must be similarly phosphorylated before their antiviral functions are apparent. Nucleoside analogs have been used for the treatment of EBV infection, and more successfully in the treatment of HIV infection (Chapter 5).

In review, each deoxynucleotide (in DNA) and ribonucleotide (in RNA) consists of three parts – 1. a nucleobase, 2. a sugar molecule (deoxyribose for DNA and ribose for RNA), and 3. phosphate (PO_4). The starting point is the nucleobase, for example, thymine. To make thymidine nucleoside, deoxyribose is added. To make thymidine deoxynucleotide, phosphate is added, by TK. Thymidine deoxynucleotide, in the form of the triphosphate, is added to growing DNA strands.

Thymidine Kinase Negative (TK Neg.) HSV Mutants

In laboratory cultures of HSV (grown in the presence of acyclovir), and also in HSV isolates from patients being treated with acyclovir, HSV mutants resistant to acyclovir have been detected. These mutants typically lack the HSV TK and are termed "TK negative" (TK neg.) mutants. Lacking the viral TK, they do not phosphorylate acyclovir to the active antiviral state, and, therefore, they are not inhibited by acyclovir.

It is emphasized that such HSV TK neg. mutants are selected by acyclovir from populations of millions of infectious HSV particles, and not that TK neg. mutants are caused by acyclovir. The very few virus particles that are TK neg. replicate in the presence of acyclovir, and, therefore, their numbers are magnified when the background of usual wild-type TK pos. HSV is inhibited by acyclovir.

Such TK neg. HSV can be easily detected in a modified plaque assay. In this assay, HSV is investigated by a plaque assay, as in Chapter 2. However, the culture medium added to plates after they are infected with HSV contains radioactive deoxythymidine nucleoside. Wild-type HSV that is TK pos. and that has the viral TK will phosphorylate the radioactive deoxythymidine nucleoside to the deoxythymidine nucleotide. This radiolabeled deoxythymidine nucleoside will be incorporated into the viral DNA and can be seen (radioactive signal) in wild-type TK pos. plaques. TK neg. HSV will not phosphorylate the radiolabeled deoxythymidine nucleoside, and label will not be incorporated into TK neg. plaques.

When x-ray film is placed over stained and dried plates, TK pos. HSV plaques will have a dark rim, the result of the exposure of x-ray film to radioactive nucleoside in the rim of plaques. Mutant TK neg. HSV will not phosphorylate the radioactive nucleoside. Therefore, TK neg. mutant HSV plaques will not appear black on the x-ray film. A mixture of wild-type HSV TK pos. and TK neg. mutant HSV are seen in Figure 8.1.[76]

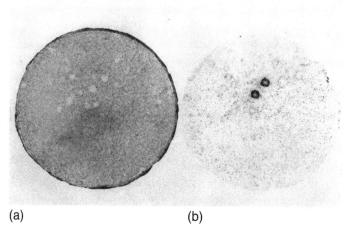

(a)   (b)

Figure 8.1 Plaque assay of a mixture of standard, wild-type TK pos. HSV and mutant TK neg. HSV. (a) The stained monolayer 4 days after infection, including one day with radioactive dT in the medium. Twenty-one HSV plaque-forming units (PFUs) are present. (b) An autoradiograph of the same plate showing two dark-rimmed plaques. HSV TK in these two wild-type TK pos. plaques incorporated radioactive deoxythymidine into the viral DNA. Plaques that did not incorporate radioactive deoxythymidine were mutant TK neg. HSV. Ninety percent of the HSV PFUs in the isolate were TK neg., and 10% were TK pos. From Westheim AI, et al. *J Am Acad Derm* 1987;**17**:875–880. Used with permission, Elsevier.

All HSV in Figure 8.1 were from the swab of a skin lesion of an immunosuppressed patient who was receiving acyclovir.

Will TK Neg. HSV Establish Latent Infections?

Several laboratories investigated TK neg. HSV to determine the possible biological importance of the viral TK gene. Mutant TK neg. HSV grew (replicated) well in most situations except one; TK neg. HSV grew poorly in nondividing cells.

Since sensory ganglion neurons in the trigeminal ganglion are the site of HSV latent infection (Chapter 5), and since these neurons are nondividing cells, investigations were performed of possible HSV latent infection with HSV TK neg. mutants. The goal was to investigate mechanisms of HSV latent infection in neurons.

In several studies, the TK neg. HSV used was selected by its ability to grow in the presence of acyclovir. In some studies, TK neg. HSV that had been molecularly constructed to be TK neg. was used. In these mutants, the TK gene in the viral DNA was removed (they are deletion mutants).

Experiments were performed as previously to investigate HSV latent infection in mouse trigeminal ganglia. As discussed in Chapter 5, during HSV latency, infectious HSV is not isolated from homogenates of latently infected ganglia but is isolated from explants of latently infected ganglia.

Results obtained with wild-type TK pos. HSV and mutant TK neg. HSV were compared and are summarized in Table 8.1.

It was concluded that HSV TK expression was important for the establishment of HSV latent infection. As noted above, HSV TK was thought important for infection of nondividing cells, and since sensory ganglion neurons are nondividing cells, the results were in keeping with that concept.

Table 8.1 Experimental trigeminal ganglion (TG) latent infection by wild-type TK pos. HSV and mutant TK neg. HSV

Virus tested	Virus was isolated from TG homogenates[1]	Virus was isolated from TG explant cultures
Wild-type TK pos. HSV	No*	Yes*
TK neg. HSV mutant no. 1	No	No**
TK neg. HSV mutant no. 2	No	No**
TK neg. HSV mutant no. 3	No	No**

* As in Table 5.1, Chapter 5, infectious virus is not isolated from tissue homogenates of latently infected ganglia but is isolated from such ganglia by explant culture procedures – a major criterion of HSV latent infection.

** Unlike results with wild-type TK pos. HSV, none of several HSV TK neg. mutant viruses was isolated from explant cultures.

In fact, this was an instance of correct data and the incorrect interpretation of data. Specifically, the data indicated that reactivation of TK neg. HSV was not detected in ganglion explants. In terms of the interpretation: Did that mean that virus was not present in ganglia or that reactivation was impaired?

Although TK Neg. HSV Does Not Reactivate from Ganglia during Latency, Is the Virus Present in Ganglia?

The laboratories of the author and of others went a step further, which altered the interpretation of the data.

In these studies, rather than investigate whether HSV could be isolated by explant culture of ganglia (the usual means to reactivate latent

HSV), determinations of whether HSV LAT (latency associated transcript) was present in latently infected trigeminal ganglion neurons were performed. As noted in Chapter 5, Table 5.1, the detection of HSV LAT is the molecular marker of HSV latent infection. Results were striking.[77,78]

In Table 8.2, HSV LAT detection results are added (fourth column) to the results of Table 8.1.

These data suggested that TK neg. mutant HSV did in fact establish latent infection (HSV LAT was detected in the typical neuron distribution), but TK neg. mutant HSV was defective for reactivation from latency (explants culture results were negative). HSV LAT detection in ganglion neurons was as frequent for TK neg. mutant HSV as for wild-type TK pos. HSV.

It was thought that the impaired reactivation of TK neg. HSV might be related to the low levels of neuronal TK, and the low levels of nucleotides such as deoxythymidine nucleotide in the trigeminal ganglion neurons (nonreplicating cells). It was thought that these low neuronal levels might not be a detriment for wild-type TK pos. HSV that has its own TK but might be limiting for mutant TK neg. HSV that does not bring its own TK.

Table 8.2 Experimental TG latent Infection by wild-type TK pos. HSV and mutant TK neg. HSV: the detection of LAT

Virus tested	Virus was isolated from TG homogenates	Virus was isolated from TG explant cultures	HSV LAT was detected in neurons during latency
Wild-type TK pos. HSV	No	Yes	Yes
TK neg. mutant no. 1	No	No	Yes
TK neg. mutant no. 2	No	No	Yes
TK neg. mutant no. 3	No	No	Yes

Note: Numbers of LAT-positive TG neurons were similar in all groups.

This hypothesis was investigated in studies to determine whether enhancing neuronal deoxythymidine nucleotide levels could overcome the impaired reactivation of TK neg. HSV.

Addition of Supplemental Deoxythymidine (dT) Nucleoside to Enhance TK Neg. HSV Reactivation

It was thought that robust HSV TK activity (present in wild-type TK pos. HSV) performed an important function in terms of reactivation of the virus in neurons, which have low levels of cellular TK and low levels of dT. It was thought that TK neg. mutant HSV did not readily reactivate from latency, because it did not have its own viral TK and because it could not call upon the minimal neuronal TK and dT levels.

It was not possible to readily enhance neuronal TK, but it was possible to enhance neuronal dT.

Toward this end, explant cultures of trigeminal ganglia latently infected with TK neg. mutant HSV were established by usual methods. However, supplemental dT nucleoside was added to the explant culture medium, in an attempt to increase dT levels in latently infected neurons.

Deoxythymidine nucleoside was added to the explant culture medium in three concentrations (three experimental groups). Two types of controls were also included, 1. usual explant medium with no supplement, 2. explant medium containing another nucleoside (deoxycytidine [dC] nucleoside). Results are shown in Table 8.3.

In Experiment 1, 200 μM dT seemed most effective, and so in Experiment 2 a larger number of animals was studied at that concentration of dT nucleoside. Results showed that supplemental dT in explant medium greatly enhanced reactivation of TK neg. HSV, in a dose-dependent manner. Reactivation was not enhanced with control dC.

Table 8.3 Reactivation of TK neg. HSV from TG explants is enhanced by supplemental dT in the culture medium

| | Number of reactivation-positive TG/number tested (% positive) Supplemental nucleoside and concentration (μM) in explant medium | | | | |
	None	dT 50 μM	dT 100 μM	dT 200 μM	dC 200 μM
Experiment 1	0/20 (0)	1/14 (7)	6/20 (30)	10/20 (50)	0/18 (0)
Experiment 2				32/37 (86)	

μM – micromolar; dC – deoxycytidine nucleoside.
Source: Data from Tenser RB et al. *J Virol* 1996;**70**:1271–1276. Used with permission, American Society for Microbiology.

As previously (Tables 8.1, 8.2), reactivation of TK neg HSV was impaired. However, supplemental dT in the explant medium greatly enhanced reactivation of TK neg. HSV.[78]

Enhanced explant culture reactivation of TK neg. mutant HSV by the use of supplemental dT supported the conclusion that HSV TK is important for reactivation of HSV from neuronal latency. It was in accord with the special environment of the large sensory ganglion neurons, which have modest dT levels.

Inhibition of Transport of dT into Sensory Ganglion Neurons

An additional experiment was then performed to further investigate the apparent enhancing effect of supplemental dT on the reactivation of TK neg. HSV from latency. In this experiment, TK neg. HSV latently infected trigeminal ganglia were again placed in explant culture with supplemental dT, as for results in Table 8.3.

However, medication that is known to inhibit the transport of nucleosides into cells, dipyridamole (DPM), was also added to the explant medium.

It was thought that since supplemental dT reversed the reactivation block of TK neg. mutant HSV (Table 8.3), preventing dT from entering cells would restore the block. Since DPM decreases passage of nucleosides (such as dT) from entering cells, it was predicted that dT-enhanced reactivation of TK neg. HSV would be blocked.

In Table 8.4, TK neg. mutant HSV reactivation from latency was impaired (0/10 positive, 0%) unless dT was added, resulting in frequent reactivation (10/10 positive, 100%). However, dT-mediated enhanced reactivation was inhibited by DPM in a dose dependent manner (56% → 0%).

Results showed that DPM restored the reactivation block of TK neg. mutant HSV, likely by impairing the passage of dT into latently infected neurons.[79]

Interestingly, DPM has been used to treat people – not for virus infections, but for other conditions, such as cardiac disease. In these patients, DPM has been used clinically to alter nucleoside transport, as

Table 8.4 Reactivation of latent TK neg. HSV is enhanced by dT, and that enhancement is blocked by DPM

| Amount of dT added | Number of reactivation-positive TG/number tested (% positive) | | |
| | Amount of DPM added | | |
	0	25 μM	50 μM
0	0/10 (0)	ND	ND
100 μM	10/10 (100%)	10/18 (56%)	0/19 (0%)

ND – not done; μM – micromolar; DPM – dipyridamole.
Source: Data from Tenser RB et al. *Antimicrob Agents Chemother* 2001;**45**:3657–3659. Used with permission, American Society for Microbiology.

it was used in the above experiment. The fact that DPM has been used in patients to decrease nucleoside transport enhances the interpretation of the DPM-TK neg. HSV results (Table 8.4).

The enhanced reactivation of TK neg. HSV from latently infected neurons by supplemental dT (Table 8.3), and the block of this reactivation by DPM (Table 8.4) supports the hypothesized importance of HSV TK expression in reactivation from neurons, probably related to the low TK and dT levels in the neurons.

Would Supplemental dT Have Any Effect on In Vivo Infection?

It is much easier to perform and interpret studies in cell culture, such as explants of trigeminal ganglia, than studies in intact animals. However, the goals of most biological studies are to extend results to individuals. With the above evidence that dT nucleoside enhanced the reactivation of mutant TK neg. HSV from latent infection of trigeminal ganglion neurons (Table 8.3), the performance of a related in vivo study in mice was planned.

In these studies mice were infected with wild-type TK pos. or with mutant TK neg. HSV, and trigeminal ganglion tissue was assayed for HSV.

Experimental group mice received dT in their drinking water, and control mice did not. In preliminary studies it was found that mice drank less water with added dT than they drank normally. When dT water was tasted, it was found that the dT made it somewhat bitter. Therefore, sugar (5% sucrose) was added to dT drinking water of mice. However, mice receiving dT in their drinking water still drank less than those that were not given dT in their water.

The amounts of water consumed, both regular tap water and water supplemented with dT and sugar is indicated in Table 8.5, as is the amount of dT consumed, calculated from the amount of water consumed.

Table 8.5 Effect of oral dT on mutant TK neg. HSV infection in mice

Virus group	Amount of water consumed per day (ml)	Amount of dT consumed per day (mg)	No. virus-positive TG/ No. tested	Ave. HSV PFU/TG
TK neg.	13.8	NA	0/8	0
TK neg.	7.3	183	8/8	2,800
TK pos.	13.0	NA	8/8	58,000
TK pos.	7.6	198	8/8	42,000

NA – not applicable, these mice did not receive any dT in their drinking water;
PFU – plaque-forming units per trigeminal ganglion.
Source: Data from Tenser RB et al. *J Virol* 1996;**70**:1271–1276. Used with permission, American Society for Microbiology.

Mice infected with wild-type TK pos. HSV and mutant TK neg. HSV were studied. Results included numbers of trigeminal ganglia with detectable HSV (No. virus-HSV positive trigeminal ganglion (TG)/No. tested) and average amounts of HSV in trigeminal ganglia (plaque-forming unit [PFU]/TG).

Observations were the following:

Under ordinary circumstances, HSV was not detected in TG of mice infected with mutant TK neg. HSV (0/8) as previously, but with dT feeding, all ganglia (8/8) were positive.

While no HSV was detected in ganglia after infection with mutant TK neg. HSV under ordinary conditions, with dT feeding, an average of 2,800 HSV PFU/ganglion were detected.

From these data, it was apparent that dT feeding enhanced mutant TK neg. HSV infection of trigeminal ganglia.[78]

There was no increase of wild-type TK pos. HSV infection, probably because this infection is maximal under usual circumstances. It is not thought that the decrease in PFUs after dT nucleoside consumption (58,000 to 42,000) is significant, but this would need be further evaluated.

While average amount of dT consumed per day was calculated, dT amount in mice was not measured, and use of other nucleosides were not studied.

In performing studies in intact animals, the intact animal is sometimes thought of as a "black box"; intact individuals are much more complicated than are cell cultures. The biochemical complexity of intact individuals sometimes leads to results in cell culture studies that cannot be replicated in intact animals. The fact that dT nucleoside supplement results were similar in intact animals as in cell culture likely enhanced the applicability of the results.

The mechanisms of HSV latency in neurons and reactivation are unclear. However, it appears that with sensory ganglion neurons being a nondividing cell type, the viral TK is important. Interestingly, it appears to be important not for the establishment of latency but for reactivation from latency. It is suggested that the since the viral TK appears to be not important for the establishment of latency, viral replication is not necessary for the establishment of latency, while it is important for the reactivation process.

Of possible importance, dT has been used to decrease cell replication in cell culture (termed "thymidine block"). In those situations, inhibition of cell replication is thought to occur when excessive deoxythymidine nucleoside results in excessive deoxythymidine nucleotide, which alters the equilibrium of other cellular deoxynucleotides. The slight decrease in wild-type TK pos. HSV replication in trigeminal ganglia may not be significant, but given the inhibition of cell replication by large amounts of dT (thymidine block), further study may be warranted.

Experimental Animal Studies

In studies of HSV latent infection performed by the author and colleagues, studies were performed with living adult mice. Although the latently infected living mice appeared to have normal behavior, and their eating, drinking, and weight were similar to uninfected mice, study of trigeminal ganglion tissues from these mice required them to be sacrificed (killed). Humane methods were used for this. In all instances, mice were anesthetized with sodium pentobarbital. When unconscious, cardiac puncture was performed, and blood was removed, resulting in death. Trigeminal ganglia (right and left) were then removed and studied for HSV latency.

Further Reading

EE Heldwein, GA Smith, eds. *Alphaherpesviruses: Molecular Biology, Host Interactions and Control*, Caister Academic Press, 2020. Book 978–1–913652–55–5, Ebook 978–1–913652–56–2

Y Xie, L Wu, M Wang, et al. Alpha-herpesvirus thymidine kinase genes mediate viral virulence and are potential therapeutic targets. *Front Microbiol* 2019;**10**:941. https://doi.org/10.3389/fmicb.2019.00941

The Future

Men willingly believe what they wish.

– Julius Caesar

That is, what one thinks will happen is closely tied to what one wishes will happen.

Antivirals

Some aspects of the future of Neurovirology and Virology are easy to predict, because of present research, for example, the development of antivirals. Since the development of acyclovir, an antiviral of specificity and safety to treat herpes simplex virus (HSV) and varicella-zoster virus (VZV), other antivirals have been developed. These have been in large part in response to the human immunodeficiency virus (HIV) pandemic. New antivirals and use of combinations of antivirals have had a great impact on decreasing HIV infections and in decreasing the occurrence of the acquired immunodeficiency disease syndrome (AIDS).

Antivirals such as remdesivir and molnupiravir showed early promise in the treatment of SARS-CoV-2 infections. Such individual antivirals may be surpassed in efficacy by combinations, such as nirmatrelvir in combination with ritonavir, and by remdesivir in combination with molnupiravir. Combinations of antivirals have been very valuable in the treatment of HIV infections and may be the future in treating other viral infections. It is likely that these are only the tip of the developing antiviral iceberg. Some antivirals are being repurposed, that is, being investigated for the treatment of viral illnesses other than the illness for which they were initially developed.

In addition, new antivirals are being developed.[80,81] As part of this, and Important for neurovirology, is the concept of the blood–brain barrier, which limits the penetration of some medications into the central nervous system.[82]

Vaccines and Antibodies

Vaccines against viral illnesses have been a success story of medicine and science (for example, poliomyelitis virus and measles virus vaccines). In some instances, such as for influenza virus, vaccines are altered to keep up with viral changes, but this changing virus has been the exception rather than the rule. SARS-CoV-2 variants have reemphasized the issue. It is likely that not only will there be new vaccine developments in the direction of multivariant control of SARS-CoV-2, but the mRNA vaccine methodologies will permit control of variants of other viruses, such as influenza.

The efficacy of the RNA vaccines developed in response to the COVID-19 pandemic has put proof to the concept of RNA vaccines.[38–40] They are likely to grow in importance not only in the prevention of many infectious illnesses but also in the treatment of noninfectious illnesses.

The use of monoclonal antibodies has been very important in the contemporary treatment of cancer. This will likely grow with developments in mRNA vaccine technology.

ANTIBODIES AS DELIVERY SYSTEMS

Antibodies are useful to inhibit targets (for example, a viruses), as discussed above, but will also likely be useful to deliver medications to targets, for example, to deliver medication to abnormal cells.

A strength of antibodies is that they are generally safe and they bind to specific protein antigens. With the use of antibodies derived from mRNA vaccines, the focus is enhanced. Antibody resulting from an mRNA vaccine is very specific in target recognition – a single site of a single protein. Could such antibody be used to deliver medication to cells, for example, to deliver antisense oligonucleotides?

An antisense DNA oligonucleotide (Chapters 3, 5) may be used to decrease an mRNA, and therefore to decrease production of an abnormal protein. However, the clinical delivery of therapeutic antisense oligonucleotides to specific cellular targets has been difficult. Use of monoclonal antibody may be a means to deliver therapeutic DNA oligonucleotides to specific abnormal cells. Then, by antisense inhibition, the oligonucleotides would inhibit the abnormal cellular mRNA and, therefore, the abnormal protein.[54,83]

Similarly, specific antibody may be useful as the delivery system for chemotherapeutic medications to cancer cells as a means of focal chemotherapy. Such focal chemotherapy would permit greater amounts of chemotherapeutics to be delivered to specific neoplastic targets and to minimize the systemic side effects of chemotherapy.

Immune Senescence

The immune system decreases in efficiency with age, an important factor in considering many illnesses, including viral infections.[17] This immune senescence is significant for the acquired immune system, particularly for T lymphocyte functions. While some B lymphocyte functions are relatively easy to measure, by measuring antibody, measuring T cell functions are more difficult.

Not too long ago, clinical T lymphocyte testing was restricted to skin tests, such as the tuberculin skin test. However, clinically useful T lymphocyte tests are becoming available, and these may be of great value in following immune system function over time – such as immune senescence.[17,84,85]

NEUROLOGICAL VIRAL INFECTIONS

Viral infections of the nervous system are often more severe in the very young and in the elderly. Comparisons of T lymphocyte functions in these groups will enhance understanding of viral pathogenesis. Shingles (herpes-zoster) occurrence due to VZV reactivation is often age related; when it occurs in young individuals, it is often related to immunosuppression. These observations may provide an important focus for research – the immune functions decreased in young individuals who are immunosuppressed and develop shingles may be similar to those in the normal elderly (with presumed immune senescence) who develop shingles.[16]

NEUROLOGICAL AUTOIMMUNE ILLNESSES

In multiple sclerosis (MS), exacerbations (relapses) decrease in frequency with age, which in this autoimmune illness may also be related to decreased immune activity with age. As is true for measuring immune parameters in immunosuppressed young and in elderly shingles patients, studies of immune parameters, particularly T lymphocyte functions in MS patients, will likely provide insights into immune senescence. Understanding of MS pathogenesis will follow.

In considering neurological autoimmune illnesses such as the Guillain-Barré syndrome and MS, if one considers that they result from an abnormal T lymphocyte response to a viral infection or vaccine, two considerations seem to arise: 1. The individual had an abnormal response to the virus (or vaccine), and it would have occurred whenever the individual was exposed to that agent. 2. The abnormal response occurred at the specific time observed because the immune system was "primed," and it might not have occurred at other times.

METHODS TO MEASURE T LYMPHOCYTE FUNCTIONS

The development of methods to quantitate T lymphocyte functions will permit the study of T lymphocytes of old versus young patients, in terms of understanding varicella-zoster shingles and MS pathogenesis. Similarly, this will permit the investigation of lymphocytes of Guillain-Barré patients to determine whether their cells continue to abnormally reactive to specific antigens, or possibly that when they developed Guillain-Barré, their cells had been "primed" to react. Factors that might "prime" the immune system may relate to epigenetics.

Epigenetics

With age, our genes are unchanged, but the expression of our genes may change. Epigenetics investigates factors that turn genes on and off. One could see how this might be important in considering change of immune function with age. The power and emphasis of epigenetics in the consideration of many illnesses are difficult to predict, but they are likely to be great.[27] Epigenetics is of importance in considering the cause as well as the treatment of cancer, such as malignant brain tumors.[86]

In MS in identical twins, the concordance is about 30–35%, suggesting a significant genetic component of the illness. That the concordance is not higher suggests an important environmental factor to which one twin had been exposed whereas the other had not. The environmental factor might have been one being infected with a virus, with disease resulting – a traditional model. Alternatively, it might have been an environmental factor that turned specific immune responsiveness on (or off), leading to the initiation of illness – an epigenetic model.

Epstein–Barr virus (EBV) infection is almost universal in MS, but most EBV-positive individuals do not develop MS.[70] There may be a genetic reason, in that the immune system of some individuals reacts aberrantly to EBV (measures of T lymphocyte functions will be important), or there may be an epigenetic reason.

The issue of MS immune-related exacerbations is similar. Are the factors that cause MS the same as the factors that cause exacerbations of MS? Again, one can speculate on epigenetic control of immune factors that turn on (or off) gene-related functions, which result in exacerbations. Measures of T lymphocyte function discussed above will permit following of at least some aspects of T cell function that are related to environmental factors and to age.[84,85]

Epidemiology

There has been great growth in epidemiological concepts in recent years, and this will likely continue. There will be undoubted growth in the polymerase chain reaction (PCR) industry. Not only will PCR testing continue to be used in many situations where individuals are clinically sick – and the infecting organism can be determined by PCR testing – but its use will be expanded in individuals who are not sick. That is, it will be used for epidemiological reasons. For example, in the next influenza epidemic/pandemic, it is likely that PCR testing of individuals who are not clinically sick will be widely performed, as in the recent COVID-19 pandemic.

The epidemiological concept of screening non-sick individuals for infectious agents will likely continue, and it will change clinical medicine, where in the past only sick individuals were tested for possible infectious agents.

PCR testing is very powerful and compelling, such as the ready identification of SARS-CoV-2 variants. This may be clinically important if variants are less sensitive to vaccines, as has been the case for some influenza virus variants.

As part of the PCR surge, however, PCR anxiety will likely be a concern. Acting on abnormal PCR positive results in clinically normal individuals – such as instituting isolation or quarantine – will be important in public health situations.

Prions and Other Atypical Agents

Prions, proteins that recruit normal proteins to become abnormal and which effect can be transmitted to other individuals, are so odd that it is difficult to predict their future. Possible are prion-like illnesses where abnormal proteins recruit normal proteins to become abnormal, but are not transmissible to other individuals. Studies of degenerative illnesses such as Alzheimer's disease, where abnormal protein accumulates, will further evaluate the occurrence of such prion-like entities. The concept of "infectious" (that is, transmissible) proteins (that is, prions) may lead to investigations of such "infectivity" of other molecules.

Philosophically, the biology of prions, viroids, and virusoids would seem to deny life form status to these agents. Simply because they replicate is not sufficient to consider them as alive. These agents are not life forms but more like toxins that replicate.[29,21]

Endogenous retroviral elements, present in the DNA of humans, also blur the separation between infectious and metabolic diseases. Many millennia ago, these RNA viruses, in the form of pro-viral DNA, became part of cellular DNA.[60] If illness results from these DNA sequences, it would likely be more appropriate to consider the illness as metabolic (due to abnormal DNA expression) than as infectious.

Such RNA retroviruses exist in humans in the form of DNA provirus sequences, and it is unclear as to benefit or harm they cause. It is likely that with antiviral developments and further understanding of viral latency, inhibition or removal of such DNA provirus sequences will be investigated.

Viral Latency

Latent virus infections may be thought of as the result of virus evolution. The DNA herpesviruses particularly have evolved mechanisms to maintain themselves in host cells for many years. With reactivation of neurotropic HSV, the human host is not usually killed, virus is produced, and this infects new hosts. And the process may repeat multiple times. In many individuals, reactivation of HSV results in asymptomatic shedding of virus, which enhances the likelihood of transmission and the establishment of new latent infections. For HSV, latent infection of nondividing sensory ganglion neurons may be close to lifelong.

Viral latency has also been well described for HIV. The latent infections established by this virus have been one of the reasons why the elimination of HIV infections have proved so difficult.

Latent infection established by HIV retrovirus is in the form of a DNA provirus. One can speculate on similarities and differences between that DNA provirus and the DNA provirus form of endogenous retroviral elements.

Two types of disparate results are likely to come from experimental studies of viral latency.[46,50] First, during latency, while viral functions are very decreased, they are not absent, and it is likely that means to alter those functions will become available, for example, through the development of antivirals. Second will be investigations of the mechanisms by which the viral genes of a latent virus modify host cells. For example, latent HSV infection of trigeminal ganglion neurons, including LAT expression, may be used as a means to investigate neurons.

It was suggested (Chapter 5) that HSV may establish latent infections of brain neurons, in addition to the well-demonstrated HSV latent infections of sensory ganglion neurons. Others have noted brainstem occurrence of HSV latency.[87] If this experimental evidence is verified and extended to humans, it would require in new considerations of human central nervous system (CNS) illnesses.

Therapeutic Viruses

Two general approaches have been utilized – using viruses to kill bacteria and cancer cells, and using viruses to bring medication into cells.

VIRUSES AS LYTIC AGENTS

The concept of using bacteriophage to infect and destroy bacteria and thereby to treat bacterial infections continues. Human bacteriophage therapy has had some use in Eastern Europe. Bacteriophage therapy may have more immediate use in treating animal and plant infections, thereby decreasing antibiotic and pesticide use.[19,88]

The idea of using viruses to kill cancer cells continues, with some modifications. Investigators have considered this concept for many years, and although it continues, it has been difficult; while some viruses replicate in and destroy rapidly growing (cancer) cells preferentially, it may be difficult to limit cell destruction to only cancer cells. And the human host often mounts an immune response against the oncolytic virus.

There has been recent evidence that such oncolytic viruses may have their oncolytic effect not simply by killing cancer cells, but by exposing infected cancer cell antigens to the immune system. Antigens that in intact cancer cells are not easily accessible to the immune system may be uncovered by the virus, permitting the immune system to then destroy the cancer cells.[89]

VIRUSES AS DELIVERY SYSTEMS

Rather than using viruses as toxins is the concept of using viruses as delivery systems. Viruses bind to and enter cells, and this concept may be more fruitful in treating human illnesses than using viruses to kill cells. Patients may be treated with a virus which carries genetic information to modify target cells, including neurons.

For example, Zolgensma® is a modified adeno-associated virus containing the human *SMN1* gene that is defective in children with spinal muscular atrophy – a lethal illness. Strikingly, the motor neurons of these children are modified by the virus-mediated delivery of the human gene.[90]

A related delivery approach has been used in cancer treatment studies, not to have virus kill cancer cells, but rather to enhance the immune response to cancer. In such studies, T lymphocytes are removed from cancer patients and infected with virus carrying information to enhance the recognition of specific antigens on cancer cells. The modified T lymphocytes are then returned to the same cancer patient and they mount a T lymphocyte-mediated attack on cancer cells.

Similar to the use of viruses to deliver information to cells is the use of "virosomes" – the membranes of viruses – containing medication to be delivered to cells. A virosome contains no viral RNA or DNA, and so there is not viral replication. The virosome concept relies on the ability of viruses to bind to and to enter cells, via their membranes and their membrane proteins.[91]

MANUFACTURED VIRUS

Philosophically/ethically this is a difficult area to consider. As discussed in Chapter 1, infectious virus has been made in the laboratory from "off the shelf" chemicals.[12] The possible issues of such laboratory creation of virus, or similarly, the modification of existing virus will it is hoped be openly discussed.

However, the synthesis of "designer" virus to accomplish tasks such as destroying bacteria or cancer cells may represent a potential benefit of virus manufacture. "Replicons," noninfectious, self-replicating RNAs, have been developed to conveniently investigate some aspects of virus pathogenesis and control.[92]

Similarly, in performing important antibody-mediated virus neutralization studies, pseudo-viruses have been constructed to facilitate testing.[93]

Post-Polio Syndrome

As a clinician with interest in disease pathogenesis, the author thinks this one of the most interesting neurological illnesses discussed.

The weakness seen with clinical poliomyelitis is due to the viral destruction of motor neurons in the spinal cord (and brainstem) that innervate muscle cells. The post-polio syndrome consists of new (worsening) weakness years after clinical polio. As introduced in Chapter 7, the new weakness is thought to be due to subclinical damage of motor neurons years previously (at the time of clinical polio), which subsequently becomes clinically manifest.

In many medical situations, antecedent events are sought to correlate with and to explain the mechanisms of clinical illnesses. The post-polio syndrome does both, as well or better than others.

First, the illness post-polio syndrome occurs after clinical polio – therefore, there is a strong correlation with a well-defined antecedent infection. Second, the mechanism of post-polio is strongly suggested – it very likely due to the prior subclinical damage to motor neurons. The post-polio syndrome strongly supports the concept of early modest neuron damage as being responsible for the development of neurological illness years later.[58]

The occurrence of the post-polio syndrome is a model of clarity of illness after a presumptive antecedent event. It also provides a target for investigations of motor neurons – specifically, what type of neuron damage occurred those years previously?

Further Reading

S Pollastro, M deBourayne, G Balzaretti, et al. Characterization and monitoring of antigen-responsive T cell clones using T cell receptor gene expression analysis. *Front Immunol* 2020;**11**:6096. https://doi.org/10.3389/fimmu.2020.609624

J Rittiner, M Moncalvo, O Ckiba-falek, B Kantor, Gene-editing technologies paired with viral vectors for translational research into neurodegenerative disorders. *Front Mol Neurosci* 2020;**13**:148. https://doi.org/10.3389/fnmol.2020.00148

T Tollefsbol, *Handbook of Epigenetics*, 3rd ed., Elsevier, 2022

References

1. Bamford DH, Burnett RM, Stuart DI. Evolution of viral structure. *Theor Popul Biol* 2002;**61**:461–470. https://doi.org/10.1006/tpbi.2002.1591

2. Gigante A, Li M, Junghänel S, et al. Non-viral transfection vectors: are hybrid materials the way forward? *Med Chem Commun* 2019;**10**:1692–1718. https://doi.org/10.1039/C9MD00275H

3. Ornatsky O, Baranov VI, Bandura DR, et al. Multiple cellular antigen detection by ICP-MS. *J Immun Meth* 2006;**308**:68–76. https://doi.org/10.1016/j.jim.2005.09.020

4. Hepp C, Shiaelis N, Robb NC, et al. Viral detection and identification in 20 min by rapid single-particle fluorescence in-situ hybridization of viral RNA. *Sci Rep* 2021;**11**:19579. https://doi.org/10.1038/s41598-021-98972-z

5. Abbasi J. The flawed science of antibody testing for SARS-CoV-2 immunity. *JAMA* 2021;**326**:1781–1782. https://doi.org/10.1001/jama.2021.18919

6. Cox NJ, Subbaraok K. Global epidemiology of influenza: past and present. *Ann Rev Med* 2000;**51**:407–421. https://doi.org/10.1146/annurev.med.51.1.407

7. Ahmed A, Oldstone MBA. Organ-specific selection of viral variants during chronic infection. *J Exp Med* 1988;**167**:1719–1724. https://doi.org/10.1084/jem.167.5.1719

8. Harvey WT, Carabelli AM, Jackson B, et al. SARS-Co-V-2 variants, spike mutations and immune escape. *Nature Rev Microbiol* 2021;**19**:409–424. https://doi.org/10.1038/s41579-021-00573-0

9. Vogel G, Kupferschmidt K. Early studies shed light on omicron's behavior. *Science* 2021;**374**:1543–1544. https://doi.org/10.1126/science.acz9878

10. Katzelnick LC, Escoto AC, Huang AT, et al. Antigenic evolution of dengue viruses over 20 years. *Science* 2021;**374**:999–1004. https://doi.org/10.1126/science.abk0058

11. Hendrix RW, Lawrence JG, Hatfull GF, Casjens S. The origins and ongoing evolution of viruses. *Trends Microbiol* 2000;**8**(11):504–509. https://doi.org/10.1016/S0966-842x(00)01863-1

12. Wimmer E. The test-tube synthesis of a chemical called poliovirus. *EMBO Rep* 2006;**7**:S3–S9. https://doi.org/10.1038/sj.embor.7400728

13. Ramirez S, Fernandez-Antunez C, Galli A., et al. Overcoming culture restriction for SARS-CoV-2 in human cells facilitates the screening of compounds inhibiting viral replication. *Antimicrob Agents Chemother* 2021;**65**:1–20. https://doi.org/10.1128/AAC.00097-21

14. Worobey M. Dissecting the early COVID-19 cases in Wuhan. *Science* 2021;**374**:1202–1204. https://doi.org/1126/science.abm4454

15. Lipsitch M, Swerdlow DL, Firelli L. Defining the epidemiology of COVID-19 – studies needed. *N Engl J Med* 2020;**382**:1194–1196. https://doi.org/10.1056/NEJMp2002125

16. Amrita J, Canaday DH. Herpes zoster in the older adult. *Infect Dis Clin North Am* 2017;**31**:811–826. https://doi.org/10.1016/j.idc.2017.07.016

17. Aw D, Silva AB, Palmer DB. Immunosenescence: emerging challenges for an ageing population. *Immunology* 2007;**120**:435–446. https://doi.org/10.1111/j.1365-2567.2007.02555.x

18. Colloca L, Barsky AJ. Placebo and nocebo effects. *N Engl J Med* 2020;**382**:554–561. https://doi.org/10.1056/NEJMra1907805

19. Principi N, Silvestri E, Esposito S. Advantages and limitations of bacteriophages for the treatment of bacterial infections. *Front Pharmacol* 2019;**10**:513. https://doi.org/10.3389/fphar.2019.00513

20. Mentha N, Clément S, Negro F, Alfaiate D. A review on hepatitis D; from virology to new therapies. *J Adv Res* 2019;**17**:3–15. https://doi.org/10.1016/j.jare.2019.03.009

21. Terry C, Wadsworth JDF. Recent advances in understanding mammalian prion structure: a mini review. *Front Mol Neurosci* 2019;**12**:169. https://doi.org/10.3389/fnmol.2019.00169

22. McCormick W, Mermel LA. The basic reproductive number and particle-to-plaque ratio: comparison of these two parameters and viral infectivity. *Virol J* 2021;**18**(1):92. https://doi.org/10.1186/s12985-021-01566-4

23. Malone B, Urakova N, Snijder EJ, et al. Structures and functions of coronavirus replication-transcription complexes and their relevance for SARS-CoV-2 drug design. *Nat Rev Mol Cell Biol* 2022;**23**:21–39. https://doi.org/10.1038/s41580-021-00432-z

24. Bonilla SL, Sherlock ME, MacFadden A, Kleft JS. A viral RNA hijacks host machinery using dynamic conformational changes of a tRNA-like structure. *Science* 2021;**374**:955–960. https://doi.org/10.1126/science.abe8526

25. Ahlquist P, Noueiry AO, Lee W-M, et al. Host factors in positive-strand RNA virus genome replication. *J Virol* 2003;**77**:8181–8186. https://doi.org/10.1128/JVI.77.15.8181-8186.2003

26. Piel FB, Steinberg MH, Rees DC. Sickle cell disease. *N Engl J Med* 2017;**376**:1561–1573. https://doi.org/10.1056/NEJMra1510865

27. Cavalli G, Heard E. Advances in epigenetics link genetics to the environment and disease. *Nature* 2019;**571**:489–499. https://doi.org/10.1038/s41586-019-1411-0

28. Galmarini CM, Mackey JR, Dumontet C. Nucleoside analogues and nucleobases in cancer treatment. *Lancet Oncol* 2002;**3**:415–424. https://doi.org/10.1016/S1470-2045(02)00788-X

29. Seley-Radke KL, Yates MK. The evolution of nucleoside antivirals: a review for chemists and non-chemists. *Antiviral Res* 2018;**154**:66–86. https://doi.org/10.1016/j.antiviral.2018.04.004

30. Varga ZV, Ferdinandy P, Liaudet L, Pacher P. Drug-induced mitochondrial dysfunction and cardiotoxicity. *Am J Physiol Heart Circ Physiol* 2015;**309**:H1453–H1467. https://doi.org/10.1152/ajpheart.00554.2015.

31. Roger AJ, Nunoz-Gomez SA, Kamikawa R. The origin and diversification of mitochondria. *Current Biol*. 2017;**27**:R1177–R1192. https://doi.org/10.1016/j.cub.2017.09.015

32. Medzhitov R. The spectrum of inflammatory responses. *Science* 2021;**374**:1070–1075. https://doi.org/10.1126/science.abi5200

33. Casanova J-L, Abel L. Mechanisms of viral inflammation and disease in humans. *Science* 2021;**374**:1080–1086. https://doi.org/10.1126/science.abj7965

34. The COVID STEROID 2 Trial Group. Effect of 12 mg vs 6 mg of dexamethasone on the number of days alive without life support in adults with COVID-19 and severe hypoxemia. *JAMA* 2021;**326**:1807–1817. https://doi.org/10.1001/jama.2021.18295

35. Balasko A, Graydon C, Fowke KR. Novel in vitro invariant natural killer T cell functional assay. *J Immunol Meth* 2021;**499**:113171. https://org/10.1016/jim.2021.113171

36. Janiaud P, Axfors C, Schmitt AM, et al. Association of convalescent plasma treatment with clinical outcomes in patients with COVID-19. *JAMA* 2021;**325**:1185–1195. https://doi.org/10.1001/jama.2021.2747

37. O'Brien MP, Forleo-Neto E, Sarkar N, et al. Effect of subcutaneous casirivimab and imdevimab antibody combination vs placebo on development of symptomatic COVID-19 in early asymptomatic SARS-CoV-2 infection. *JAMA* 2022;**327**:432–441. https://doi.org/10.1001/jama.2021.24939

38. Cohn BA, Cirillo PM, Murphy CC, et al. SARS-CoV-2 vaccine protection and deaths among US veterans during 2021. *Science* 2022;**375**:331–336. https://doi.org/10.1126/science.abm0620

39. Marks PW, Gruppuso PA, Adashi EY. Urgent need for next-generation COVID-19 vaccines. *JAMA* 2023;**329**:19–20. https://doi.org/10.1001/jama.2022.22759

40. Goel RR, Painter MM, Apostolidis SA, et al. mRNA vaccines induce durable memory to SARS-CoV-2 variants of concern. *Science* 2021;**374**(6572):abm0829. https://doi.org/10.1126/science.abm0829

41. Gonzalez DC, Nassau DE, Khodamoradi K, et al. Sperm parameters before and after COVID-19 mRNA vaccination. *JAMA* 2021;**326**:273–274. https://doi.org/10.1001/jama.2021.9976

42. Blumenthal KG, Robinson LB, Camargo CA Jr, et al. Acute allergic reactions to mRNA COVID-19 vaccines. *JAMA* 2021;**325**:1562–1565. https://doi.org/10.1001/jama.2021.3976

43. Shimabukuro TT, Cole M, Su JR. Reports of anaphylaxis after receipt of mRNA COVID-19 vaccines in the US – December 14, 2020 – January 18, 2021. *JAMA* 2021;**325**:1101–1102. https://doi.org/10.1001/jama.2021.1967

44. Oster ME, Shay DK, Su JR, et al. Myocarditis cases reported after mRNA-based COVID-19 vaccination in the US from December 2020 to August 2021. *JAMA* 2022;**327**:331–340. https://doi.org/10.1001/jama.2021.24110

45. van Kammen MS, de Sousa DA, Poli S, Cordonnier C, et al. Characteristics and outcomes of patients with cerebral venous sinus thrombosis in SARS-CoV-2 vaccine-induced immune thrombotic thrombocytopenia. *JAMA Neurology* 2021;**78**:1314–1323. https://doi.org/10.1001/jamaneurol.2021.3619

46. Cohen JI. Herpesvirus latency. *J Clin Invest* 2020;**130**:3361–3369. https://doi.org/10.1172/JCI136225

47. Feldstein LR, Tenforde MW, Friedman KG, et al. Characteristics and outcomes of US children and adolescents with multisystem inflammatory syndrome in children (NIS-C) compared with severe acute COVID-19. *JAMA* 2021;**325**:1074–1097. https://doi.org/doi:10.1001/jama.2021.2091

48. Spudich S, Nath A. Nervous system consequences of COVID-19. *Science* 2022;**375**:267–269. https://doi.org/10.1126/science.abm2052

49. Singer EJ, Sueiras MV, Commins D, Levine A. Neurologic presentations of AIDS. *Neurol Clin.* 2010;**28**:253–275. https://doi.org/10.1016/j.ncl.2009.09.018

50. Julg B, Dee L, Ananworanich J, et al. Recommendations for analytical antiretroviral treatment in HIV research trials-report of a consensus meeting. *Lancet HIV.* 2019;**6**:e259–e268. https://doi.org/10.1016/S2352-3018(19)30052-9

51. Fugl A, Andersen CL. Epstein-Barr virus and its association with disease: a review of relevance to general practice. *BMC Fam Pract* 2019;**20**(1):62. https://doi.org/10.1186/s12875-019-0954-3

52. Antinone SE, Smith GA. Retrograde axon transport of herpes simplex virus and pseudorabies virus: a live cell comparative analysis. *J Virol* 2010;**84**:1504–1512. https://doi.org/10.1128/JVI.02029-09

53. Dugal-Tessier J, Thirumalairajan S, Jain N. Antibody-oligonucleotide conjugates: a twist to antibody-drug conjugates. *J Clin Med* 2021;**10**(4):838. https://doi.org/10.3390/jcm10040838

54. Chaudhuri A, Kennedy PGE. Diagnosis and treatment of viral encephalitis. *Postgrad Med J* 2002;**78**:575–583. http://dx.doi.org/10.1136/pmj.78.924.575

55. Chadwick DR. Viral meningitis. *Brit Med Bull* 2005;**75–76**:1–14. https://doi.org/10.1093/bmb/ldh057

56. Price HE, Hogrefe WR. Detection of West Nile virus (WNV)-specific immunoglobulin M in a reference laboratory setting during the 2000 WNV season in the United States. *Clin Diag Lab Immunol* 2003;**10**:764–768. https://doi.org/10.1128/CDLI.10.5.764–768.2003

57. Tyler KL. Acute viral encephalitis. *N Engl J Med* 2018;**379**:557–566. https://doi.org/10.1056/NEJMra1708714

58. Bridgens R, Sturman S, Davidson C. Post polio syndrome – polio's legacy. *Clin Med* 2010;**10**:213–214. https://doi.org/10.7861/clinmedicine.10-3-213

59. Griffin DE. Measles virus persistence and its pathogenesis. *Curr Opin Virol* 2020;41:46–51. https://doi.org/10.1016/j.coviro.2020.03.003

60. Fitzgerald B, Boyle C, Honein MA. Birth defects potentially related to zika virus infection during pregnancy in the United States. *JAMA* 2018;**319**:1195–1196. https://doi.org/10.1001/jama.2018.0126

61. Racicot K, Mor G. Risks associated with viral infections during pregnancy. *J Clin Invest* 2017;**127**:1591–1599. https://doi.org/10.1172/JCI87490

62. Stocking C, Kozak CA. Murine endogenous retroviruses. *Cell Mol Life Sci* 2008;**65**:3383–3398. https://doi.org/10.1007/s00018-008-8497-0

63. Lasky T, Terracciano GJ, Magder L, et al. The Guillain-Barre syndrome and the 1992–1993 and 1993–1994 influenza vaccines. *N Engl J Med* 1998;**339**:1797–1802. https://doi.org/10.1056/NEJM199812173392501

64. Ben David SS, Potasman I, Rahamim-Cohen D. Rate of recurrent Guillain-Barré syndrome after mRNA COVID-19 vaccine BNT162b2. *JAMA Neurol* 2021;**78**:1409–1411. https://doi.org/10.1001/jamaneurol.2021.3287

65. Deisenhammer F, Zetterberg H, Fitzner B, Zettl UK. The cerebrospinal fluid in multiple sclerosis. *Front Immunol* 2019;**10**:726. https://doi.org/10.3389/fimmu.2019.00726

66. Tenser RB, Sommerville KW, Mummaw JG, Frisque RJ. Isolation of JC virus capsomer-like structures from progressive multifocal leukoencephalopathy brain. *J Neurol Sci* 1986;**72**:243–254. https://doi.org/10.1016/0022-510X(86)90012-2

67. Cortese I, Reich DS, Nath A. Progressive multifocal leukoencephalopathy and the spectrum of JC virus-related disease. *Nat Rev Neurol* 2020;**17**:37–51. https://doi.org/10.1038/s41582-020-00427-y

68. White MK, Khalil L. Pathogenesis of progressive multifocal leukoencephalopathy-revisited. *J Infect Dis* 2011;**203**:578–586. https://doi.org/10.1093/infdis/jiq097

69. Leray E, Moreau T, Fromont A, Edan G. Epidemiology of multiple sclerosis. *Rev Neurol (Paris)* 2016;**172**:3–13. https://doi.org/10.1016/j.neurol.2015.10.006

70. Bjornevik K, Cortese M, Healy BC, et al. Longitudinal analysis reveals high prevalence of Epstein-Barr virus associated with multiple sclerosis. *Science* 2022;**375**:296–301. https://doi.org/10.1126/science.abj8222

71. Maitland MT, Frederiksen JL. Vaccines and multiple sclerosis: a systemic review. *J Neurol* 2017;**264**:1035–1050. https://doi.org/10.1007/s00415-016-8263-4

72. Sormani MP, Tintorè M, Rovaris M, et al. Will Rogers phenomenon in multiple sclerosis. *Ann Neurol* 2008;**64**:428–433. https://doi.org/10.1002/ana.21464

73. McGuire LI, Peden AH, Orrú CD, et al. RT-QuIC analysis of cerebrospinal fluid in sporadic Creutzfeldt-Jakob disease. *Ann Neurol* 2012;**72**:278–285. https://doi.org/10.1002/ana.23589

74. Eccleston PA, Funa K, Heldin C-H. Neurons of the peripheral nervous system express thymidine phosphorylase. *Neurosci Lett* 1995;**192**:137–141. https://doi.org/10.1016/0304-3940(95)11622-4

75. Bitter EE, Townsend MH, Erickson R, et al. Thymidine kinase through the ages: a comprehensive review. *Cell Biosci* 2020;**10**(1):138. https://doi.org/10.1186/s13578-020-00493-1

76. Westheim AI, Tenser RB, Marks JG Jr. Acyclovir resistance in a patient with chronic mucocutaneous herpes simplex infection. *J Am Acad Derm* 1987;**17**:875–880. https://doi.org/10.1016/S0190-9622(87)70272-2

77. Chen S-H, Pearson A, Coen DM, Chen S-H. Failure of thymidine kinase-negative herpes simplex virus to reactivate from latency following efficient establishment. *J Virol* 2004;**78**:520–523. https://doi.org/10.1128/JVI.78.1.520-523.2004

78. Tenser RB, Gaydos A, Hay KA. Reactivation of thymidine kinase-negative herpes simplex virus is enhanced by nucleoside. *J Virol* 1996;**70**:1271–1276. DOI:https://doi.org/10.1128/jvi.70.2.1271-1276.1996

79. Tenser RB, Gaydos A, Hay KA. Inhibition of herpes simplex virus latency by dipyridamole. *Antimicrob Agents Chemother* 2001;**45**:3657–3659. https://doi.org/10.1128/AAC.45.12.3657-3659.2001

80. Owen DR, Allerton CMN, Anderson AS, et al. An oral SARS-CoV-2 M^pro inhibitor clinical candidate for the treatment of COVID-19. *Science.* 2021;**374**:1586–1593. https://doi.org/10.1126/science.abl4784

81. Sourimant J, Lieber CM, Aggarwal M, et al. 4′-fluorouridine is an oral antiviral that blocks respiratory syncytial virus and SARS-CoV-2 replication. *Science* 2022;**375**:161–167. https://doi.org/10.1126/science.abj5508

82. Richardson PJ, Ottaviani S, Prelle A, Stebbing J, Casalini G. CNS penetration of potential anti-COVID-19 drugs. *J Neurol* 2020;**267**:1880–1882. https://doi.org/10.1007/s00415-020-09866-5

83. Hammond SM, Aartsma-Rus A, Alves S, et al. Delivery of oligonucleotide-based therapeutics: challenges and opportunities. *EMBO Mol Med* 2021;**13**(4):e13243. https://doi.org/10.15252.emmm.202013243

84. Reus B, Caserta S, Larsen M, et al. In-depth profiling of T-cell responsiveness to commonly recognized CMV antigens in older people reveals important sex differences. *Front Immunol* 2021;**12**:707830. https://doi.org/10.3389/fimmu.2021.707830

85. Zollner A, Watschinger C, Rössler A, et al. B and T cell response in SARS-CoV-2 vaccination inn health care professionals with and without previous COVID-19. *EBioMedicine* 2021;**70**:103539. https://doi.org/10.1016.jbiom.2021.103539

86. Suter RK, Rodriguez-Blanco J, Ayad NG. Epigenetic pathways and plasticity in brain tumors. *Neurobiol Dis* 2020;**145**:105050. https://doi.org/10.1016/j.nbd.2020.105060

87. Doll JR, Thompson RL, Sawtell NM. Infectious herpes simplex virus in the brain stem is correlated with reactivation in the trigeminal ganglia. *J Virol* 2019;**93**(8):e02209-18. https://doi.org/10.1128/JVI.02209-18

88. Lin DM, Koskella B, Lin HC. Phage therapy: an alternative to antibiotics in the age of multidrug resistance. *World J Gastrointest Pharmacol Ther* 2017;**83**:162–173. https://doi.org/10.4292/wjgpt.v8.i3.162

89. Melcher A, Harrington K, Vile R. Oncolytic virotherapy as immunotherapy. *Science*. 2021;**374**:1325–1326. https://doi.org/10.1126/science.abk3436

90. Klotz J, Rocha CT, Young SD, et al. Advances in the therapy of spinal muscular atrophy. *J Ped* 2021;**236**:13–20. https://doi.org/10.1016/j.jpeds.2021.06.033

91. Kumar V, Kumar R, Jain VK, Nagpal S. Preparation and characterization of nanocurcumin based hybrid virosomes as a drug delivery vehicle with enhanced anticancerous activity and reduced toxicity. *Sci Rep* 2021;**11**(1):368. https://doi.org/10.1038/s41598-020-79631-1

92. Ricardo-Lax I, Luna JM, Thao TTN, et al. Replication and single-cycle delivery of SARS-CoV-2 replicons. *Science* 2021;**374**:1099–1106. https://doi.org/10.1126/science.abj8430

93. Muik A, Lui BG, Wallisch A-K, et al. Neutralization of SARS-CoV-2 omicron by BNT162b2 mRNA vaccine-elicited human sera. *Science* 2022;**375**:678–680. https://doi.org/10.1126/science.abn7591

Index

active immunization (vaccines), defined, 18
acyclovir, 63
adaptive immune system
  after immune cell education, 68
  antibody testing, 78–83
  B cells (B lymphocytes), 75–78
  human white blood cells, 71–72
  T cells (T lymphocytes), 72–75
adenosine triphosphate (ATP), 65
animal studies, 180–93
animal viruses and human infection, 23–24
antibody
  3-dimensional structure of, 61–62
  future of, 195–96
  and immunization, 18
  immunoglobulin (Ig) lymphocytes, 73
  testing response duration, 82–83
  and viral infections, 17–18
antibody testing
  antibody response duration, 82–83
  ELISA, 81
  immunoglobulin (Ig) lymphocytes, 78–79
  immunohistochemistry, 80
  lateral flow technology, 81
  neutralizing antibody titer, 81–82
  plaque reduction method, 40–43
  titer, 79
antigenic drift, 21
antigenic shift, 21

antigens, T cells (T lymphocytes), 73–74
antisense inhibition
  defined, 54–55
  RNA virus, 56–57
  in situ hybridization, 117
anti-viral medications
  acyclovir, 63
  azidothymidine (AZT), 65
  background, 18
  development of, 63
  didanosine, 65
  future of, 194–95
  lamivudine, 64
  molnupiravir, 64
  nirmatrelvir, 64
  remdesivir, 63–64
anti-viral vaccines
  commonly used, 84
  fertility vaccine issues, 88
  goal of, 84
  history of, 83–84
  immunosuppressed patients, 88–89
  issues, 87–88
arboviruses
  bunyavirus, 129
  dengue fever virus, 130
  flavivirus, 130
  togavirus, 130
  transmission, 129
  yellow fever virus, 130
  Zika virus, 130

Asian flu
history of, 19
viral cause of, 20
atypical agents
future of, 200–1
types of, 32
autosomal dominant genetic
abnormality, 60
autosomal recessive genetic
abnormality, 60
axoplasmic transport
botulism, 108
pathogenesis, 107
rabies, 108–9
tetanus, 108
azidothymidine (AZT)
HIV (human immunodeficiency
virus), 65
mitochondrial myopathy, 65–66

B cells (B lymphocytes)
adaptive immune system, 75
background, 73, 75–77
monoclonal antibody, 77–78
polyclonal antibody, 77
bacteriophages, 30–31
birth defects, 135–36
BK virus infection, 157–58
Black Death (1348–1352), 19
blood–brain barrier (BBB), 152
blood type and genes, 58
blot hybridization
nomenclature, 16
northern, 10–11
Southern, 10–11
western, 15
botulism, 108
bunyavirus, 129

cancer, virus causing, 5
cell surface proteins and viral
infections, 5–6
Central Dogma
process summary, 57–58
transcription, 55–56
translation, 57

Central Dogma (synthesis), 46–47
cerebrospinal fluid (CSF)
blood brain barrier (BBB), 152
IgG index, 152–55
IgG measurement, 151–52
infections, 151
lumbar puncture, 150–51
physiology of, 150
clinical medicine, 26
codon, 57
complementation
DNA, 48
immune system, 71
RNA, 51
COVID-19
asymptomatic possibilities, 29
cause of, 20
cytokine storm, 69–70
monoclonal antibody, 78
mortality from, 19
origin of, 24–25
T cells (T lymphocytes), 74–75
vaccine side effects, 91–92
Western SARS-CoV-2, 84
Creutzfeldt–Jakob disease, 172–73,
176–78
Creutzfeldt–Jakob disease, iatrogenic
transmission, 175–76
cystic fibrosis, 60
cytokine storm
COVID-19, 69–70
SARS-CoV-2, 70
cytokines
innate immune system, 69
multiple sclerosis, 70
cytomegalovirus (CMV), 135

data interpretation, virus detection
versus data, 9
PCR (polymerase chain reaction),
7–9
dengue fever virus, 130
deoxynucleotides (DNA)
nucleosides into, 51–52
virus, 48
didanosine, 65

direct method of
    immunohistochemistry, 12–13
DNA replication
  background, 46
  Central Dogma, 46–47
  human, 47–50
  as template for mRNA, 50
  virus, 50
dorsal root ganglion virus pathology,
    105–7
double helix (DNA), 47

efficacy of treatment, 28
electron microscopy, 16–17
ELISA (enzyme-linked
    immunosorbent assay), 14–15, 81
encephalitis
  case report, 132–33
  herpes simplex virus (HSV),
    133–35
  paraneoplastic (autoimmune), 132
  viral, 131
endogenous retroviruses
  as atypical agent, 32
  defined, 136–37
  evolution, 22
epidemiology
  and clinical medicine, 25–26
  future of, 199–200
  group emphasis, 26
  placebo and nocebo effects, 28–29
  probability and statistics, 27
epigenetics, 198–99
epitope, 17
Epstein–Barr virus (EBV), 101–3

flavivirus, 130

gain of function, 25
genes
  blood type and, 58
  defined, 58
genetic abnormalities
  autosomal dominant, 60
  autosomal recessive, 60
  X-linked recessive, 60

girus, 16
Guillain-Barré syndrome, 145,
    146–47, 149

hepatitis medications, 64
herpes B virus, 127–28
herpes simplex virus (HSV)
  acyclovir, 63
  animal viruses, 115
  asymptomatic possibilities,
    29–30
  birth defects, 135–36
  DNA synthesis, 50
  experimental animal studies,
    180–93
  infection criteria, 110–11
  latent infections, 114–15
  reactivation speculation,
    139–40
  in situ hybridization, 112–14
  trigeminal system virus pathology,
    109–12
  viral pathogenesis, 103–4
  viral plaque assays, 35–40
  zoonotic virus infections, 126–27
herpes simplex virus (HSV)
    encephalitis, 133–35
HIV (human immunodeficiency
    virus)
  anti-viral medications, 64–65
  mitochondrial myopathy,
    65–66
  viral pathogenesis, 98–101
Hong Kong flu
  history of, 19
  viral cause of, 20
human genome, 47
human herpesvirus 6/7, 127
human immunodeficiency virus
    (HIV), 128
human polyoma viruses
  BK virus infection, 157–58
  JC virus infection, 158–60
human T cell lymphotrophic virus
    type 1 (HTLV-1), 128
Huntington's disease, 60

hybridization
  northern blot hybridization, 10–11
  pros and cons, 53–54
  in situ, 112–14, 117–20
  Southern blot hybridization, 10–11

IgG measurement, 152–55
immune system
  adaptive, 68, 71–78
  case study, 143–45
  complement, 71
  innate, 69–70
  interferons, 70
  overview, 68
  senescence, 196–97
immunoglobulin (Ig) lymphocytes
  B cells (B lymphocytes), 75–77
  types of, 73
immunohistochemistry methods of
    virus detection, 80
in situ hybridization
  antisense inhibition, 117
  herpes simplex virus (HSV),
    112–14
  varicella-zoster virus (VZV),
    117–20
incubation period, 96
indirect method of
    immunohistochemistry, 13
infectious human virus classification,
    123–24
infectious virus categories, 122–23
infectious virus measurement, 34–43
influenza virus
  antigenic shift and antigenic drift,
    21–22
  principle proteins, 20
  as RNA virus, 19–20, 51
influenza virus pandemic
    (1918–1919)
  history of, 19
  viral cause of, 20
innate immune system
  cytokine storm, 69–70
  cytokines, 69
  protein polymorphism, 69

interferons
  multiple sclerosis and, 70
  types of, 70

JC virus infection, 158–60

Kuru, 172–73

latent infections
  background, 95–96
  defined, 6
  endogenous retroviruses, 138–39
  future of, 201–2
  neurological viral illness, 156–57
  reactivation speculation, 139–40
  types of, 119
  viral latency versus latent period,
    96
latent period, 96
lateral flow technology method of
    virus detection, 15
long COVID-19, 98
lumbar puncture, 150–51
Lyme disease, 129
lymphocytes
  B cells (B lymphocytes), 73, 75–78
  defined, 72
  immunoglobulin (Ig) lymphocytes,
    73
  NK (natural killer cells), 72–73
  T cells (T lymphocytes), 72, 73–75
lysogeny, 95
lytic infections
  defined, 6, 30
  future of, 202
  overview, 94–95

mad cow disease, 175
manufactured virus, 203
measles virus
  and human infection, 23
  as RNA virus, 51
MERS (Middle East respiratory
    syndrome)
  cause of, 20
  remdesivir, 63–64

messenger RNA (mRNA)
  DNA template for, 50
  as synthesis template, 46
  transcription, 55–56
mitochondria
  defined, 65
  as endosymbionts, 65
  from mother, 66
mitochondrial myopathy, 65–66
molecular mimicry, 146–47
molnupiravir, 64
monoclonal antibody
  B cells (B lymphocytes), 77–78
  cancer treatment, 78
  defined, 18
  process of, 75–77
multiple sclerosis
  clinical observations, 162
  cytokines and, 70
  demyelination, 160–61
  epidemiology, 162–64
  exacerbations of, 164–65
  interferon treatment, 70
  National Vaccine Injury
    Compensation Program, 165–66
  pseudo-exacerbations, 165
  treatment, 168
  vaccines and, 165–66
myelitis, 149

National Vaccine Injury
    Compensation Program, 165–66
nervous system
  cerebrospinal fluid (CSF), 155
  inflammatory illness, 149–50
  physiology of, 148–49
  viral infections, 124–30
neurological autoimmune illness
  future of, 197
  Guillain-Barré syndrome, 145
  multiple sclerosis, 160–68
neurological viral illness
  future of, 197
  human polyoma viruses, 157–60
  latent infections, 156–57
  post-polio syndrome, 171

prion illnesses, 172–79
  SSPE (subacute sclerosing
    panencephalitis), 155–56
  Will Rogers phenomenon, 168–70
neurovirology
  background, 142–43
  HSV experimental animal studies,
    180–93
  post-infectious neurological
    illness, 146–47
neutralizing antibody titer, 81–82
nirmatrelvir, 64
NK (natural killer cells), 72–73
nocebo effect, 28
northern blot hybridization, 10–11
nucleosides, 51–52

obligate intracellular organisms,
    viruses as, 3
oncolytic virus, 31

paraneoplastic encephalitis, 132
passive immunization (vaccination),
    18
PCR (polymerase chain reaction)
  data interpretation, 7–9
  methodology, 52–53
  SARS-CoV-2, 7
  target nucleic acid, 7
peroxidase-antiperoxidase
    immunohistochemistry, 13
placebo effect, 28
plaque reduction method, 40–43
poliomyelitis virus
  overview, 125–26
  synthesis of, 24
  vaccine development, 86
  vaccines for, 86
polyclonal antibody
  B cells (B lymphocytes), 77
  defined, 17
polycystic kidney disease, autosomal
    dominant genetic abnormality,
    60
positron emission tomography
    (PET), 168–70

post-infectious neurological illness, 146–47
post-polio syndrome
  future of, 204–5
  overview, 171
prion neurological illnesses
  Creutzfeldt–Jakob disease, 172–73
  Creutzfeldt–Jakob disease, iatrogenic transmission, 175–76
  Kuru, 172–73
  mad cow disease, 175
  non-transmissible, 178–79
  scrapie, 173
prions, 32, 138, 174–75
protein polymorphism
  innate immune system, 69
  sickle cell disease, 59
  viral infection resistance, 58–59
protein structure, 61
protein synthesis
  Central Dogma, 57
  genes and, 58–59

rabies, 108–9, 124–25
remdesivir, 63–64
reverse transcription, 51
ribonucleotides (RNA)
  nucleosides into, 51–52
  virus, 51
RNA replication
  background, 46
  virus, 50–51
RNA vaccines, 92–93
RNA virus
  influenza virus, 19–20
  poliomyelitis virus, 24
rubella virus, 135

SARS (severe acute respiratory syndrome)
  antigenic shift and antigenic drift, 21
  cause of, 20
SARS-CoV-2,
  antibody testing, 78–79
  antigenic shift and antigenic drift, 21–22

anti-viral medications, 63–64
anti-viral vaccines, 84
B cells (B lymphocytes), 77
blood type O and, 59
cytokine storm, 70
data interpretation, 7–9
origin of, 24–25
PCR (polymerase chain reaction), 7, 52–53
post-immunization infection, 89–90
pregnancy immunization, 88
as RNA virus, 51
viral pathogenesis, 97–98
viral plaque assays, 40
viral variants, 90–91
scrapie, 173
sickle cell disease
  autosomal recessive genetic abnormality, 60
  protein polymorphism, 59
slow virus infection, 138–39, 155–56
smallpox virus
  history of, 83–84
  and human infection, 23
Southern blot hybridization, 10–11
SSPE (subacute sclerosing panencephalitis), 155–56

T cells (T lymphocytes)
  COVID-19, 74–75
  foreign protein antigens, 73–74
  future of testing methods, 198
  measurement difficulties, 73
  testing difficulty, 74
  tuberculosis skin testing, 74
  types of, 72
target DNA, 52–53
tetanus, 108
therapeutic viruses
  bacteriophages, 30–31
  oncolytic virus, 31
  virus vectors, 30
titer, antibody
  defined, 79
  neutralizing, 81–82

togavirus, 130
toxoid vaccines, 87
transcription
    Central Dogma, 55–56
    RNA virus, 56–57
transfection, 5
translation, 57
trigeminal ganglia system virus
        pathology, 105–7
trigeminal system virus pathology,
        109–12
tropism, 3
tuberculosis skin testing, 74

vaccines
    development of, 20
    future of, 195
varicella-zoster virus (VZV), 117–20,
        127
variolation, 83
viral encephalitis, 131
viral infections
    antibody and, 17–18
    antiviral medications, 18
    and cancer, 5
    versus living virus, 6–7
    process of, 5–6
    replication and, 4–5
    transfection, 5
    tropism, 3
viral meningitis, 131–32
viral pathogenesis
    axoplasmic transport, 107–9
    defined, 94
    Epstein–Barr virus (EBV), 101–3
    herpes simplex virus (HSV), 103–4
    HIV (human immunodeficiency
        virus), 98–101
    latent infections, 95–96
    lytic infections, 94–95
    SARS-CoV-2, 97–98
    trigeminal ganglia system virus
        pathology, 105–7
viral plaque assays
    herpes simplex virus (HSV),
        35–40

plaque reduction method, 40–43
    SARS-CoV-2, 40
viral protein detection methods
    direct method, 12–13
    ELISA (enzyme-linked
        immunosorbent assay), 14–15
    indirect method, 13
    label importance, 12
    lateral flow technology, 15
    peroxidase-antiperoxidase
        immunohistochemistry, 13
    western blot, 15
viral replication
    infection and, 4–5
    as living organism evidence, 3
virion, 16
viroids, 32, 137–38
virology
    antigenic shift and antigenic drift,
        21–22
    evolution, 22–24
    future of, 33
    history of, 18–20
    recombination events, 24
    therapeutic viruses and atypical
        agents, 30–32
virus, noninfectious, 3
virus delivery systems, 203
virus detection methods
    electron microscopy, 16–17
    northern blot hybridization, 10–11
    PCR (polymerase chain reaction),
        7–9
    Southern blot hybridization,
        10–11
    viral protein methods, 12–15
virus vectors, 30
viruses
    asymptomatic possibilities, 2
    defined, 1–2
    structure of, 2–3
viruses as living organisms
    controversy around, 2
    duration on hard surfaces, 4
    versus infectious viruses, 6–7
    obligate intracellular organisms, 3

viruses that infect the nervous system
  arboviruses, 129–30
  herpes B virus, 127–28
  herpes simplex virus (HSV), 126–27
  herpes simplex virus (HSV)
    encephalitis, 133–35
  human herpesvirus 6/7, 127
  human immunodeficiency virus
    (HIV), 128
  human T cell lymphotrophic virus
    type 1 (HTLV-1), 128
  measles virus, 128–29
  paraneoplastic encephalitis, 132
  poliomyelitis virus, 125–26
  varicella-zoster virus (VZV), 127
  viral encephalitis, 131
  viral meningitis, 131
  zoonotic virus infections, 125–30
viruses that infect the nervous
    system, birth defects
  cytomegalovirus (CMV), 135
  herpes simplex virus (HSV), 135–36
  rubella virus, 135
  Zika virus, 136

viruses that infect the nervous
    system, endogenous
    retroviruses
  anatomy, 136–37
  latent infections, 138–39
  prions, 138
  slow virus infection, 138–39
  viroids, 137–38
  virusoids, 137
virusoids
  as atypical agent, 32
  inflammatory illness, 137

western blot virus detection, 15
Will Rogers phenomenon, 168–70

X-linked recessive genetic
    abnormality, 60

yellow fever, 19
yellow fever virus, 130

Zika virus, 130, 136
zoonotic virus infections, 124–30